Hospital Pharmacy

Edited by

Martin Stephens

BPharm, MSc, MRPharmS, MCPP

Chief Pharmacist
Southampton University Hospitals NHS Trust
Southampton, UK

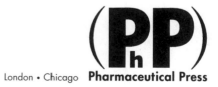

London • Chicago **Pharmaceutical Press**

Published by the Pharmaceutical Press
Publications division of the Royal Pharmaceutical Society of Great Britain

1 Lambeth High Street, London SE1 7JN, UK
100 South Atkinson Road, Suite 206, Grayslake, IL 60030-7820, USA

© Pharmaceutical Press 2003

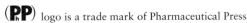 logo is a trade mark of Pharmaceutical Press

First published 2003

Text design by Barker/Hilsdon, Lyme Regis, Dorset
Typeset by Mathematical Composition Setters Ltd, Salisbury, Wiltshire
Printed in Great Britain by TJ International, Padstow, Cornwall

ISBN 0 85369 502 4

A catalogue record for this book is available from the British Library

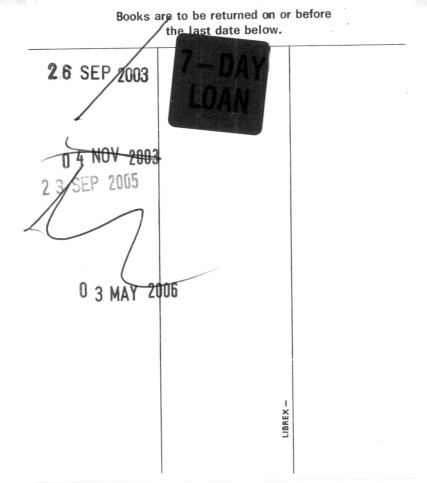

Contents

Preface   xi
About the editor   xiii
Contributors   xv
Abbreviations   xvii

Introduction   xix
Hospital pharmacy   xix
Documents key in hospital pharmacy's development   xxi
Conclusion   xxii
References   xxiii
Further reading   xxiii

1   Hospital pharmacy within the National Health Service   1
History   1
The new NHS until 2002   3
Evolution of primary care organisations   5
Scotland   6
Wales   6
Northern Ireland   6
Shifting the Balance of Power   7
The NHS Plan   7
NHS hospital trusts   8
Pharmacy's place in a trust   10
Pharmacy staff   13
The future   14
References   15
Further reading   15

2   Purchasing medicines   17
Background   17
History   18
Hospital procurement and the application of EU legislation   20
The strengths of the contracting process   22
The organisation of hospital contracts   22
Systems and processes   24
Recent changes   25

Local arrangements 25
The future 27
References 27
Further reading 28

3 Medicines supply 29
History 30
Current practice 31
The future 42
References 44
Further reading 45

4 Technical services 47
History 48
Repackaging (prepacking, assembly) 51
Non-sterile manufacture 54
Sterile manufacture 57
Aseptic preparation 60
Education and training for hospital technical services 67
Health and safety and environmental issues 68
The future 68
Acknowledgement 70
References 70
Further reading 71

5 Quality assurance 73
The NHS quality agenda and the role of the QA pharmacist 74
The aims of NHS pharmaceutical quality assurance services 76
Development, issue, implementation and monitoring of standards
    and guidance 78
Quality assurance and quality control of medicines 78
Quality assurance of pharmacy services 79
Quality assurance of aseptic services 80
Quality audit 81
Advisory services 81
Research and development 82
Testing piped medical gas installations 82
Training of pharmacy staff 82
Defective medicines 83
Laboratory services 83
Environmental monitoring services 86
The future 87
References 88
Further reading 90

6   Medicines information   91
History   91
Structure and activities   92
Aims and strategy   93
Roles and skills   95
Ethics and legal issues   95
Clinical governance and risk management   99
Customers/users   104
Activities   105
Specialist information services   113
Information resources   114
Information technology   115
Staffing and training   116
The future   118
Conclusion   118
References   119
Further reading   120

7   Clinical pharmacy services   121
Definition of medicines management   121
Ward pharmacy   121
History   122
Clinical pharmacy   124
Pharmaceutical care   125
Activities that are components of the delivery of pharmaceutical care
    in hospitals   126
Services linked to clinical specialities   136
Moving into prescribing   143
The future   145
References   146
Further reading   150

8   Strategic medicines management   151
Clinical risk   151
Financial risk   151
History   152
Strategic medicines management in practice   154
External influences on strategic medicines management in hospitals   165
Conclusion   167
References   168
Further reading   169

9   Managing risk   171
Controls assurance   171

Quality in the NHS   174
Risk management   178
Conclusion   184
References   184
Further reading   186

10   **Community services pharmacy**   187
History   187
What are community health services?   190
Advice   190
Supply   192
Information   195
Education and training   195
Monitoring safe practices with medicines   196
Supporting the implementation of public health programmes   196
School nursing and school vaccination programmes   196
Residential and nursing home – inspection and training   197
Supporting intermediate and continuing care services for the elderly   198
Support for people with learning disabilities   199
Working with other agencies   199
The future   200
References   201
Further reading   202

11   **Information technology**   203
History   203
Electronic data interchange   204
Stock control systems   205
Electronic patient record   206
Automation   208
Conclusion   209
References   209
Further reading   210

12   **Research and development**   211
Definitions   211
History   212
Project design   214
The future   220
References   221
Further reading   222

13   **Education and training**   223
History   223

The present day   225
Management and leadership   229
The future   229
References   230
Further reading   231

14   Managing services   233
Pharmacy management   233
Business planning   236
Preparing a business case   237
Budget management   238
Benchmarking   240
Staff management   243
Conclusion   251
References   251
Further reading   251

15   Support organisations   253
Hospital Pharmacists Group (HPG)   253
British Pharmaceutical Students Association (BPSA)   254
The College of Pharmacy Practice (CPP)   254
United Kingdom Clinical Pharmacy Association (UKCPA)   258
European Society of Clinical Pharmacy (ESCP)   259
Centres for Pharmacy Postgraduate Education   261
Guild of Healthcare Pharmacists (GHP)   264
References   265
Further reading   265

Index   267

Preface

Hospital Pharmacy gathers texts on the key features of pharmaceutical services provided within and from hospital-based pharmacies in the UK. The focus will fall on the National Health Service (NHS), although, within a different context, patient needs in private hospitals are not dissimilar. The book gives an introduction to the service, of benefit to pre-registration graduates and to undergraduates. It also aims to be of benefit to recently qualified pharmacists undertaking further studies or whilst gaining wider training in rotational roles. Technicians in training or seeking broad insight into hospital pharmacy have also been considered in developing the book. Additionally I wish to echo the comments from Allwood and Fell's *Textbook of Hospital Pharmacy* who hoped its contents provided information and discussion useful to the experienced pharmacist in this country and elsewhere [1]. Indeed, anyone wishing to gain an understanding of pharmacy practice in UK hospitals will, I hope, find the book of considerable help.

The book has been structured on functional lines, that is, there are chapters on purchasing, supply, clinical services, medicines information and so on. To some extent these boundaries are artificial and functions can be blurred; to give an example, the clinical responsibilities of a pharmacist ensuring the safe preparation and supply of total parenteral nutrition are not easily split into separate roles. However, there is a need to group in some way so a pragmatic approach has been taken. Chapters have been included on education and training, research and development and on information technology; these impact on each of the other functions but they are also areas where special skills are required and indeed where specialist posts have been developed.

Each chapter attempts to describe the ground to be covered, providing definitions where these assist. The historical context is set, followed by the detail of how hospital pharmacy is currently practised. Authors have also commented on any changes expected in the subject being discussed. Some key texts are suggested as further reading to support each chapter.

I hope readers will gain benefit from the wide range of experience the authors have brought to the text and that the book is one which can be revisted regularly by hospital pharmacy staff.

Martin Stephens
October 2002

1.   Allwood M C, Fell J T. *Textbook of Hospital Pharmacy*. Oxford: Blackwell, 1980.

About the editor

Martin Stephens graduated with a Bachelor of Pharmacy degree from the University of Nottingham in 1979, completing a preregistration year in South Warwickshire hospitals in 1980. He then worked in hospital pharmacy services in the West Midlands region, undertaking roles in medicines information, clinical services, community services, education and training, and dispensary management. In 1989 he became Chief Pharmacist at Wolverhampton Hospitals where he worked until 1997, during which period he also undertook two periods of additional general management responsibility.

Martin has been Chief Pharmacist at Southampton University Hospitals NHS Trust since 1997 and Clinical Director for Clinical Support since 1998. He became a member of the College of Pharmacy Practice in 1986 and completed a masters in health economics and management at Sheffield University in 2000. Martin also served on the Hospital Pharmacist Group Committee from 1995 to 2001.

Contributors

Elaine Bartlett BPharm, MRPharmS
Principal Pharmacist, Selly Oak Hospital, Birmingham, UK

John W Barnett FRPharmS
Hospital Pharmacy Consultant, Worcester, Worcestershire, UK

Ian M Beaumont BSc, MRPharmS
Director of Quality Control, North West Region, Stockport, UK

Trevor Beswick BSc, MSc, CPPE
Head of Medicines Management, Bristol South and West PCT, Bristol, UK

Lynne Bollington DipClinEdMed, MRPharmS
All Wales Principal Pharmacist – Education, Training and Personal
Development, Cardiff, UK

**Damian Child BPharm, MSc, DipClinPharm, DipHospPharmMangt,
MCPP, MRPharmS**
Director of Pharmacy, Salford Royal Hospitals NHS Trust, Salford, UK

Jonathan Cooke BPharm, PhD, MRPharmS
Director of Pharmacy, South Manchester University Hospitals NHS
Trust, Manchester, UK

Keith Farrar BSc, MPharm, MCPP, MRPharmS
Chief Pharmacist, The Wirral Hospital NHS Trust, Wirral, UK

Ray Fitzpatrick BSc, PhD, MRPharmS
Clinical Director of Pharmacy, The Royal Wolverhampton Hospitals
NHS Trust, Wolverhampton, UK

Peter Golightly BSc, DLP, MRPharmS
Director Trent MI Services, Leicester, UK

Sarah Hiom BPharm, PhD, MRPharmS
All-Wales Research and Development Pharmacist, St Mary's Pharmacy Unit, Penarth, South Glamorgan, UK

Philippa Jones MPharm, MRPharmS, ACPP
Acting Head of Pharmacy, North Manchester Healthcare NHS Trust, Manchester, UK

Pippa Roberts BSc, DipClinPharm, CertMangt
Chief Pharmacist, Chelsea & Westminster Hospital, London, UK

David Samways BPharm, MRPharmS
Pharmacy Services Director, East Gloucestershire NHS Trust, Cheltenham, Gloucestershire, UK

Graham Sewell BPharm, PhD, MRPharmS, CBiol, MIBiol, CChem, MRSC
Professor of Clinical Pharmacy and Pharmacy Practice, Department of Pharmacy and Pharmacology, University of Bath, Bath, UK

Peter Sharott BSc, MRPharmS
Regional Pharmaceutical Adviser (Secondary Care), NHSE London, UK

Ann Slee BPharm, MSc, DipClinPharm, MRPharmS
Principal Pharmacist, The Wirral Hospital NHS Trust, Wirral, UK

Martin Stephens BPharm, MSc, MRPharmS, MCPP
Chief Pharmacist, Southampton University Hospitals NHS Trust, Southampton, UK

Howard Stokoe BSc, MRPharmS
Pharmaceuticals Procurement Executive, NHS Supply Agency, Reading, UK

Beth Taylor OBE, BSc, MRPharmS
Community Pharmacy Services Team Manager, Southwark Primary Care Trust, London, UK

Mark Tomlin BPharm, MSc, MRPharmS
Directorate Pharmacist, Critical Care, Southampton University Hospitals NHS Trust, Southampton, UK

Jayne Wood BSc, MPhil, MCPP, MRPharmS
Associate Director of Diagnostics and Clinical Support, Pennine Acute Trust, Bury, UK

Abbreviations

A&E	Accident and Emergency
ACCP	American College of Clinical Pharmacy
ADR	adverse drug reaction
AIC	Analytical Information Centre
AIDS	acquired immunodeficiency syndrome
ARSAC	Administration of Radioactive Substances Advisory Committee
ASTMS	Association of Scientific, Technical and Managerial Staff
ATOs	assistant technical officers
BPSA	British Pharmaceutical Students Association
CDs	controlled drugs
CG	clinical governance
CHI	Commission for Health Improvement
CHS	community health services
CIR	critical incidence report
CIVAS	Centralised Intravenous Additive Services
CNST	clinical negligence scheme for trusts
COSHH	Control of Substances Hazardous to Health
CPD	continuing professional development
CPP	College of Pharmacy Practice
CPPE	Centre for Pharmacy Postgraduate Education in England
CSM	Committee on Safety of Medicines
CSP	community service pharmacist
CTC	clinical trial certificate
CTX	clinical trial exemption certificate
DCA	direct-to-consumer advertising
DDX	doctor or dentist exemption certificate
D&T	drug and therapeutics
D&TC	drugs and therapeutics committees
DGHs	district general hospitals
DoH	Department of Health
EAHP	European Association of Hospital Pharmacists
EDI	electronic data interchange
EMEA	European Agency for the Evaluation of Medicinal Products
EP	electronic prescribing
ePACT	electronic prescribing analyses and cost
EPR	electronic patient record
EPSA	European Pharmaceutical Students' Association
ESCP	European Society of Clinical Pharmacy
EU	European Union
FAQs	frequently asked questions
FCE	finished consultant episode

GHP	Guild of Healthcare Pharmacists
GMP	good manufacturing practice
GP	general practitioner
GPA	government procurement agency
HEPA	high-efficiency particulate air
HIV	human immunodeficiency virus
HPG	Hospital Pharmacists Group
HPLC	high-performance liquid chromatography
HSDUs	hospital sterilising and disinfecting units
HSR	health service research
ICP	integrated-care pathway
IM	intramuscular
IPR	individual performance review
IT	information technology
IV	intravenous
IVN	intravenous nutrition
KNMP	Royal Dutch Association for the Advancement of Pharmacy
LHG	local health group
LIMS	Laboratory Information Management Systems
LREC	local research and ethics committee
MBA	Masters in Business Administration
MCA	Medicines Control Agency
MI	medicines information
MIS	medicines information service
MM	Medicines Management
MMM	Modern Materials Management
MREC	multicentre research ethics committees
MSF	Manufacturing, Science and Finance
MTO	medical technical officer
NCSC	National Care Standards Commission
NeLH	National Electronic Library for Health
NHS	National Health Service
NHSC	National Horizon Scanning Centre
NHSE	NHS executive
NICE	National Institute for Clinical Excellence
NICPPET	Northern Ireland Centre for Postgraduate Pharmaceutical Education and Training
NPA	National Pharmaceuticals Association
NPC	National Prescribing Centre
NPSA	National Purchasing and Supply Agency
NPSG	National Pharmaceutical Supplies Group
NVQ	National Vocational Qualification
OJEC	*Official Journal of the European Communities*
OTC	over-the-counter
PACT	prescribing analyses and cost
PaSA	Purchasing and Supply Agency
PCA	patient-controlled analgesia
PCG	primary care group
PCO	primary care organisation

PCT	primary care trust
PGDs	patient group directions
PHATE	pharmacy tendering evaluation
PIANA	Pharmacy In A New Age
PIGs	practice interest groups
PILs	patient information leaflets
PITS	Pharmaceutical Interlaboratory Testing Scheme
PL	product licence
PODs	patients' own drugs
POMs	prescription-only medicines
PPR	pharmacy practice research
PPRS	Pharmaceutical Price Regulation Scheme
PQE	Post Qualification Education
PVC	polyvinyl chloride
RCT	randomised controlled trial
RHAs	regional health authorities
QA	quality assurance
QC	quality control
R&D	research and development
RPSGB	Royal Pharmaceutical Society of Great Britain
SAFF	Service and Financial Framework
SCOPE	Steering Committee on Pharmacy Postgraduate Education
SCPPE	Scottish Centre for Post Qualification Pharmaceutical Education
SLA	service level agreement
SOHHD	Scottish Office Home and Health Department
TASS	Technical, Administrative and Supervisory Staffs
TDM	therapeutic drug level monitoring
TPN	total parenteral nutrition
TQM	total quality management
TSET	Technical Specialist Education and Training
UKAS	United Kingdom Accreditation Service
UKMI	UK Medicines Information
UKMIPG	UK Medicines Information Pharmacists Group
UKCPA	United Kingdom Clinical Pharmacy Association
UKCPRS	UK Standard Clinical Products Reference Source Project
VDUs	visual display units
WCPDP	Welsh Committee for Professional Development in Pharmacy
WCPPE	Welsh Centre for Postgraduate Pharmaceutical Education
WTEs	whole-time-equivalent posts

Introduction

Martin Stephens

Hospital pharmacy

It may be tempting to say that definitions and boundaries 'used to be clearer' at some point in the past, blaming the blurring of identities on the postmodern world. For hospital pharmacy, I think such a claim would mislead. Whilst there would be common agreement on certain activities being 'pharmacy' undertaken in what is clearly a 'hospital', there has never been a definitive, universally accepted description of what hospital pharmacy comprises. Neither has there been a clear demarcation of what falls outside hospital pharmacy's remit. For example, does hospital pharmacy include dispensing for hospital outpatients? In Scotland, and in some English trusts, dispensing for hospital outpatients is not part of the service provided by the hospital pharmacy. Do the community pharmacies dispensing for hospital outpatients (FP10HPs in England) consider themselves part of the hospital pharmacy service? What of hospitals that employ pharmacists who give direct advice to general practitioners – is it hospital pharmacy when based in the hospital building and primary care when based in the surgery? Certainly, the arrival of primary care trusts and the development of care trusts could further blur the boundaries. Lack of a precise definition for hospital pharmacy is not unique to the UK. In his book on hospital pharmacy in the USA, Hassan uses a 1951 American definition which describes a service under the direction of a pharmacist 'from which all medications are supplied', 'where special prescriptions are filled', where injectables '*should* be prepared', where supplies are '*often* stocked' – clearly room for some variation [1].

Having acknowledged that the edges may be fuzzy, we can note that there have been attempts to describe key functions and responsibilities of hospital pharmacy services. In 1955 the Linstead report on the hospital pharmaceutical service included a statement of the key functions [2]. These included dispensing, promoting economy in usage and 'instructing or advising those who handle the material provided'. The buzzwords of the current provision of health care and some of the current roles may be missing, but the report contains the essential principles on which hospital pharmacy still works. In the 1980s the English Regional Pharmaceutical Officers developed standards for the service: the second edition (1989) contained 28 areas of practice [3]. These standards describe what is expected if a specified service is present; the standards mention purchase, supply, clinical and drug information amongst others. Similarly, the Chief Administrative Pharmaceutical Officers in Wales drew up a standards document, which was developed into a document describing the constituents of a comprehensive pharmaceutical service and which supported audit against the standards set [4].

Taking a patient's perspective, hospital pharmacy can be described as: providing medicines, information and advice to inpatients and outpatients, as well as to the health professionals and others giving them health care. There is, of course, much more to hospital pharmacy services than the patient sees. Ensuring the appropriate purchase of medicines, establishing safe systems to store and supply medicines, decision-making on formularies, budgetary planning and many other roles surround the provision of care. In A *Spoonful of Sugar*, the Audit Commission makes clear its expectation that pharmacy should be a patient-centred service, closely linked to the rest of the clinical team [5]. Reducing risk to patients and reducing financial risk to organisations are described as key pharmacy functions. Inevitably, to achieve these functions, education and training, management, quality assurance, research and application of information technology are required to underpin the service.

In summary, hospital pharmacy is about ensuring that medicines are available and are used safely and effectively by informed patients and professionals both within the environs of a hospital and beyond. The service has moved a long way in this direction since the Noel Hall Report of 1970 [6]. The report stated: 'the pharmacist can no longer be regarded as only a dispenser of medicines ... he has also to co-operate with medical and nursing staff in securing the most effective safe and economical use of drugs'. The report was an important landmark for hospital pharmacy. Later chapters should make clear that at least some of the potential identified in 1970 has been achieved. The progress made means pharmacists and other pharmacy staff are key members of the 21st-century hospital health care team, contributing over a broad range of duties towards effective patient care.

Documents key in hospital pharmacy's development

The NHS and pharmacy have changed significantly over the last 30 years. For hospital pharmacy I believe five key documents are worthy of mention in this introductory chapter. Two have already been mentioned; all will crop up again in later chapters. The list is not comprehensive for pharmacy and does not attempt to include some important NHS policy documents that have had a major impact on the service; chapter 2 will touch on some of these.

① The Noel Hall Report (1970)

This was the report of a committee established in 1968 to review pharmaceutical services in the NHS. In addition to the quotation given above – pharmacy isn't just dispensing – the report identified the need for cooperation between departments to avoid a fragmented ineffective service, for a good career structure and for good training for pharmacists and their staff. The 1974 reorganisation of the NHS (see chapter 1) opened the way for implementation of cooperation on a district and area basis. Training opportunities and specialised posts have developed well since that time, although staff shortages can still disrupt [6].

② The Nuffield Report (1986)

This was a report to the Nuffield Foundation following an inquiry of a committee led by Sir Kenneth Clucas that ranged across the whole of pharmacy practice and the profession. The recommendations included the statement 'clinical pharmacy should be practised in all hospitals'. Movement of tasks to support staff and the need for additional resources were identified. Cooperation on 'drug information', manufacturing and quality control was commended, as it was in the Noel Hall Report. More research, pharmacists reporting adverse drug reactions, 24-hour cover, increased pay for basic grades and better career structures for technicians were amongst the other recommendations [7].

③ *The Way Forward* health circulars (1988)

Issued by the various home-country NHS bodies, these circulars stated clearly the need for effective clinical pharmacy services throughout the NHS. Though implementation and resourcing were left to local decision-making, these circulars gave the service considerable impetus and the opportunity for hospital pharmacy mangers to develop their clinical services [8].

Pharmacy in the Future (2000)

This document was made pharmacy's piece of *The NHS Plan* [9]. Meeting the needs of patients, getting the most from medicines and using the pharmacist's expertise were central themes. Much of the document deals with pharmacy's community role, but reengineering hospital pharmacy services to deliver the best standards was emphasised – practices already seen in some hospitals. 'One-stop dispensing' (see chapter 3), self-administration and pharmacists working on admission wards are given as examples of good practice. Pharmacist prescribing was proposed as a way of using pharmacists' skills and giving a better service for patients [10]. For Scotland *The Right Medicine: A Strategy for Pharmaceutical Care in Scotland*, issued in 2002, lays out the strategic direction for pharmacy; its recommendations include self-administration schemes and medication review before discharge [11]. In Wales the Task and Finish Group on Prescribing gave advice on a range of issues related to prescribing and medication [12].

A Spoonful of Sugar (2001)

The Audit Commission document *A Spoonful of Sugar* accompanied a major audit exercise undertaken across hospital pharmacy departments. It dealt with medicines management in NHS hospitals, pointing out the hazards of medicines as well as their potential benefits. Patient safety and financial stability were identified as at risk where medicines management is not done well. Amongst the 33 recommendations were: to invest in electronic prescribing and automated dispensing, to ensure enough pharmacy staff for clinical pharmacy, to ensure all hospital staff are trained for their roles with medicines, to introduce one-stop dispensing and to use original packs. The document was an important endorsement of the role of pharmacy in the NHS [5].

Conclusion

These documents have been part of hospital pharmacy's progress; some of the themes recur and have not yet seen full implementation. The NHS and pharmacy in the NHS will not become static. The development of pharmacist prescribing, the increased use and usefulness of information technology and robotics and the development of specialist practitioners will mean that hospital pharmacy continues to progress. The need for the pharmacist and the pharmacy technician with their support team to help plan for, organise and deliver health care is great. I hope this book assists in that process by informing and preparing them for their roles.

References

1. Hassan W E. *Hospital Pharmacy*, 5th edn. Philadelphia: Lea and Febiger, 1986.
2. Standing Pharmaceutical Advisory Committee. Ministry of Health. *Report of the Sub-committee on the Hospital Pharmaceutical Service*. London: HMSO, 1955.
3. Regional Pharmaceutical Officers' Committee. *Standards for Pharmaceutical Services in Health Authorities in England*, 2nd edn. 1989.
4. Morgan D, Way C, eds. *Standards for Pharmaceutical Services in Health Authorities and Trusts in Wales*. Directors of Pharmaceutical Public Health and Chief Pharmacists' Committee (Wales) 1997.
5. Audit Commission. *A Spoonful of Sugar – Medicines Management in NHS Hospitals*. London: Audit Commission, 2001.
6. Hall N, chair. *Report of the Working Party Investigating the Hospital Pharmaceutical Service*. London: HMSO, 1970.
7. Clucas K, chair. *Pharmacy: The Report of a Committee of Inquiry Appointed by the Nuffield Foundation*. London: The Nuffield Foundation, 1986.
8. Department of Health. *The Way Forward for Hospital Pharmaceutical Services*. HC 88 (54). London: Department of Health, 1988. Also WHC 88 (66) (Wales) 1988 and 1988 (GEN) 32 in Scotland.
9. Department of Health. *The NHS Plan*. London: The Stationery Office, 2000.
10. Department of Health. *Pharmacy in the Future*. London: Department of Health, 2000.
11. Scottish Executive. *The Right Medicine: A Strategy for Pharmaceutical Care in Scotland*. Edinburgh: Scottish Executive, 2002.
12. National Assembly for Wales. *Report of the Task and Finish Group on Prescribing*. Cardiff: National Assembly for Wales, 2000.

Further reading

Audit Commission. *A Spoonful of Sugar – Medicines Management in NHS Hospitals*. London: Audit Commission, 2001.
Clucas K, chair. *Pharmacy: The Report of a Committee of Inquiry Appointed by the Nuffield Foundation* (Chapter 4). London: The Nuffield Foundation, 1986.
Department of Health. *Pharmacy in the Future*. London: Department of Health, 2000.

1

Hospital pharmacy within the National Health Service

Martin Stephens

The National Health Service (NHS) is a large and complex organisation responsible for the great majority of health care in the UK. It has a workforce of over one million and employs over 4000 pharmacists. This chapter will summarise the changes in NHS organisation from inception through to *The NHS Plan* [1] and *Shifting the Balance of Power* [2], before describing the typical NHS acute hospital trust structure. Having established the context it will describe the range of staff and roles within hospital pharmacy and exemplify career pathways typical for pharmacists in the NHS.

History

The NHS became a reality in the UK on 5 July 1948. It provided general practitioner (GP) and hospital care, free at the point of delivery on the basis of need. There was optimism that good health care would mean a healthier nation and thus a decreasing demand for health spending. This hope has not been fulfilled, with demographic change, increased expectation and the ability to do more meaning an ever-increasing demand for funding. An early response to this increase was the introduction of fees – prescription charges and dental treatments. However, the majority of care has remained free, with the NHS funded from general taxation. A renewal of the commitment to this approach followed the Labour party's election victory in 2001.

    Twenty-eight years after its formation, the first of the major reorganisations of the NHS in England took place; the 1974 change was preceded by changes in the service in Wales and Scotland. In England, a triple-layer NHS was established above the individual hospitals. Regional health authorities (14 in all) were made responsible for area health authorities (90) which in turn managed district management teams (206). Within area health authorities, a parallel structure of family practitioner committees overseeing general practice was established. This change gave the opportunity to organise pharmacy services beyond individual hospitals – creating cooperation in an area pharmaceutical service along the lines of the Noel Hall Report [3].

In 1982, one of the three layers was removed – area health authorities were disbanded. This left regional and district health authorities. District health authorities managed hospitals and certain aspects of primary care – district nursing and health visitors, for example, but not general practice. There was a move to general management in 1984 following the Griffiths Report [4]. This change resulted in a reduction of the influence of senior medical and nursing staff within hospitals, with decision-making moving to general managers. The system included a chain of management from the centre via region district to the hospital, with unit general managers in each hospital being directly accountable to district general managers. However, the problems of overspending and of waiting lists remained, often resulting in emotive articles in the media. A further reorganisation was inevitable.

The Conservative government introduced the NHS and Community Care Act in 1990. It opened the way for an internal market and cutting the direct management line by introducing purchasers and providers of care. This split meant that responsibility for delivering health care (the operations, the clinics and so on) and ordering health care (setting the targets for how many operations, asking for certain new services) could be divided between different organisations that no longer had a direct management link. Contracts would be agreed between a purchaser and a provider for the level of care to be available. Talk of money following the patient and of competition between providers (hospitals, for example) became the norm. Hospitals and community services could become trusts – self-managing organisations within the NHS. By 1995 all hospitals, community health services and ambulance services had become trusts. Trusts had more local control to allow them to work within the 'market' and to arrange their own finances.

General practices could become fundholding, responsible for their prescribing budget, arranging and paying for elective surgery (planned work such as hernia repairs and hip operations) and for practice staff. Though never a true 'market', there were opportunities for GPs to change the hospital to which they referred patients. Fundholding continued to develop and by 1995 could include responsibility for all the care of a local population – arranging contracts for emergency as well as elective care. The fundholding system was criticised as creating a two-tier service (50% of GPs were included by 1997), with those patients not in fundholding practices 'left behind' and having poorer access to care. The internal market was criticised for creating a whole raft of invoicing and activity counting.

In 1996 a further change was made in the NHS structure: the English regional health authorities were replaced by regional offices of the NHS executive (NHSE), the government's civil service body 'running' the NHS. The NHSE regional offices were headed by regional directors and had leads for various services. Pharmaceutical advice was provided by regional advisors.

In 1997, a Labour government was elected with a commitment to 'put right' the NHS. The internal market was to be abolished but with no return to line management controls from the centre. A 'third way' of partnership and collaboration was to be brought in. A white paper *The New NHS: Modern, Dependable* set out the revised structure [5]. A purchaser/provider-like split was to stay, as were hospital trusts. However, fundholding was to be abolished, replaced by primary care groups which could evolve to primary care trusts. The Health Act 1999 brought these changes into place. In addition to these structural changes, the issues of quality of care and of health inequalities and reducing avoidable deaths were raised in *A First Class Service* [6] and *Our Healthier Nation* [7]. Modernising the service and providing additional investment were set out as key goals in *The NHS Plan*, published in July 2000 [1].

Different levels of care are defined in Table 1.1.

The new NHS until 2002

For England the Secretary of State for Health has responsibility for the NHS and for leading the Department of Health. In Scotland the NHS is a devolved responsibility; the Scottish parliament has legislative power and the minister for health and community care is responsible for the service. In Wales the National Assembly has responsibility for the NHS. Within the Welsh Assembly government, the Health and Social Services Secretary is lead for the service. A similar pattern applies in Northern Ireland but here personal social services and health care are integrated and led by the chair of the health and social services committee of the assembly.

The Department of Health in England seeks to improve the health of the nation through its role of allocating resources, setting policy, monitoring implementation and ensuring accountability. The objectives are to promote good health, and to provide effective health and social

Table 1.1   Defining levels of care

Level of care	Definition
Self-care	Health needs are met by patients in their own home setting, possibly with advice from external sources such as a community pharmacy or NHS Direct
Primary care	Health care is provided by general practitioners, practice and district nurses, community pharmacists, opticians, dentists or therapists in the home or local health care setting
Secondary care	Health care is provided in a hospital or specialist setting, normally accessed via primary care referral, although direct-access services are included. A wide range of specialities exists, including general medicine, orthopaedics, general surgery, therapies and diagnostic services
Tertiary (and higher) care	Health care is provided in a hospital or specialist setting of a more complex or specialised nature; referrals are often made by secondary care doctors. Tertiary centres usually have larger catchment areas than secondary centres and may work on a regional basis. Liver transplantation, neurosurgery and, less common cancer treatments exemplify this

care. The Department also oversees the Medicines Control Agency and the Medical Devices Agency, responsible for the licensing and control of medicines and medical devices respectively.

The NHSE is led by the Chief Executive of the NHS (a civil servant) and is the management body of the NHS. There were eight regional offices: eastern, London, northern and Yorkshire, north-west, south-east, south-west, Trent and west Midlands. A key responsibility was the performance management of trusts and health authorities, ensuring that waiting lists and financial targets were achieved. Larger capital schemes were controlled by regional offices, such as information technology projects, new building or major equipment requiring regional office approval.

The next layer was the health authority, which was responsible for arranging health care for the local population. Key tasks were agreeing a local health improvement programme (priorities for local developments/health improvement), ensuring that waiting-list targets were achieved and promoting public health. Following the publication of *The NHS Plan* [1], health authorities led local modernisation work.

Within each health authority primary care became organised within primary care organisations (PCOs), either as groups or as trusts. This replaced fundholding and was set out as a four-stage process in *The New NHS: Modern, Dependable* [5]. A steady move along the four-step process was expected, but this was hastened by the 2002 changes described below. PCOs were responsible for between around 50 000 and 250 000 people in their local areas. Typically, 20–30 GP practices were grouped together within a PCO. GPs and nursing staff, together with social services representatives, lay and health authority representatives, would run the primary care group (PCG). Around 480 PCOs came into existence on 1 April 1999.

Evolution of primary care organisations

The four stages identified were:

1.   Primary care group level 1: PCG responsible together with the health authority for commissioning care for the local population. PCG remains part of the health authority.
2.   Primary care group level 2: PCG remains part of the health authority structure but with a devolved responsibility for commissioning and arranging resources for care and prescribing.
3.   Primary care trust (PCT): A PCT is an independent NHS trust which is responsible for commissioning care and managing resources, including prescribing budgets. More specialised care is commissioned on a wider basis than with the PCT.
4.   Primary care trust: In addition to commissioning, the PCT can provide services to the local population, including community health services (district nursing, for example) and community hospitals.

A further development of PCO is the establishment of care trusts, where health and social care are included, similar to the Northern Ireland model.

The 'new NHS' saw the terminology of the market removed. Service agreements replaced contracts, purchasing was replaced by commissioning. A change with particular relevance for pharmacy was made: PCOs were to have a unified budget for their commissioning and prescribing. Whilst this had already been the case within fundholding, non-fundholding prescribing was, in effect, a non-cash-limited fund, although many attempts to control spending had been made. This unified budget would mean that growth in prescribing spend could undermine a health authority's or PCT's ability to arrange (and pay for) the hospital care required for its local population. Effective management of prescribing budgets would take on increased importance.

The provision of health care in the community that did not move into PCT remained the responsibility of 'provider' trusts. The organisation of these and of the acute trusts did not significantly alter with the 1999 changes. They remained self-governing NHS organisations providing a range of services, funded, in the main, via their service agreements with health authorities and PCTs. Performance management by the NHSE became increasingly important, and waiting-list numbers and waiting times were closely monitored.

Scotland

The management executive is responsible for the strategic overview of the NHS in Scotland, setting policy and monitoring performance. Health boards (15 in total) have a role in agreeing health improvement programmes for their local populations and for commissioning both hospital and community health services. Provider organisations are the acute trusts, community trusts and the ambulance service, which is run by the special health board, the Scottish Ambulance Service. Fundholding has been replaced by GPs working together locally, although practices can work outwith these cooperatives.

Wales

Five health authorities are responsible for the NHS within Wales. Local health groups (LHGs, 22 in total) work as part of the health authorities helping to commission health care and to manage prescribing and other NHS budgets. NHS trusts provide health care on a similar basis to those elsewhere in the UK. In November 2001, after a consultative exercise, a revised structure for the NHS in Wales was announced. Three regional offices (north Wales, mid with west Wales, south with east Wales) will be created as the strategic leads for the service, replacing the five health authorities. They will have a performance management role. LHGs will be replaced by local health boards. These changes are expected to be implemented in 2003.

Northern Ireland

There is much closer working between health and social care in Northern Ireland than in Britain. The four health and social service boards work in a similar way to health authorities in England (pre-2002) but with the addition of a social care remit. They commission services for their local population from the 20 or so health and social service provider organisations.

Shifting the Balance of Power

Further significant changes to the structure of the NHS in England were identified in the document *Shifting the Balance of Power Within the NHS: Securing Delivery* [2], followed by *Shifting the Balance of Power Within the NHS: The Next Steps* [8]. These documents also deal with issues beyond structure, but only the 2002 NHS changes will be described here.

On 1 April 2002 all PCOs became PCTs. Many boundary changes and some mergers had occurred over the 3 years of PCG and PCT existence. PCTs have taken on the responsibilities previously held by health authorities, including commissioning health care for their population. The old health authorities were disestablished in April 2002 and new larger health authorities were formed – 28 in all – typically with responsibility across more than one English county. In October 2002, these formally became strategic health authorities. These strategic health authorities have a performance management role and take on the duties for capital programmes held previously by NHSE regional offices. March 2003 will see the final abolition of the regional offices; the NHS in England will be overseen by four Directorates of Health and Social Care.

The NHS Plan

The NHS Plan, A Plan for Investment, a Plan for Reform was published in July 2000 [1]. It was produced after a wide consultation and it clearly restated the core NHS values whilst arguing the need for reform alongside significant investment. Redesign around the needs of the patient was a recurring phrase. Many targets for change on both broad and detailed levels are included but some central themes run throughout the document:

- Reduced waiting times, for example, no more than a 6-month wait for an operation, to be achieved by 2005.
- National standards to see good care everywhere; best practice spread.
- More patient and user involvement in the NHS.
- Cooperation with the private sector; working more closely with social services.
- Breaking the demarcation barriers between professions, including allowing nurses and pharmacists to prescribe.

To achieve the modern NHS, investment to increase the numbers of doctors, nurses, therapists, scientists and others was highlighted, as was the need to develop leadership in the NHS. *Pharmacy in the Future* was the document dealing with the specific issues relating to pharmacy playing its part in the NHS for the future [9].

NHS hospital trusts

NHS hospital trusts do not have one simple organisational pattern. There are certain requirements that are standard and similarities in how they work. Table 1.2 details the various types of trust.

NHS hospital trusts are self-governing bodies within the NHS. Each trust has a board comprising the executives of the trust and a

Table 1.2   Provider trusts

Type of trust	Definition
Acute hospital trusts	One or more hospitals providing various types of secondary and tertiary care. They are usually multispeciality but can be single-speciality. Children's services may be provided within an acute trust alongside adult services, or from a specialised trust
Teaching hospital trusts	Like acute hospitals, but linked to a university medical school and providing a significant teaching component. Research also plays an important part in the trust and university's business. Teaching trusts usually have a significant proportion of regionally based specialised services
Community trusts	Providing community-based services such as district nursing and podiatry, possibly including acute community hospitals. These have been absorbed into primary care trusts
Combined trusts	Acute and community services provided from one organisation
Mental health and learning disability trusts	Specialist trusts providing community, secondary and specialist services for these client groups. Hospital beds and home-based services will be provided
Ambulance trusts	Ambulance services, typically arranged on a county-wide basis

group of non-executives; the board has a non-executive chair. The executives are officers of the trust, usually full-time staff with a management responsibility. The non-executives are lay members of the board with a limited time commitment to their NHS role. The non-executives have a role in ensuring that the trust meets its obligations as a public body, and in providing advice and support to the executive. A patient representative is expected to be a requirement of future trust board arrangements. The executive members of the board are typically the chief executive, the medical director, the nursing director, the finance director plus one other executive. The fifth executive can be a general manager (deputy chief executive, for example) or a human resources lead for the trust. A director of planning and, increasingly, of modernisation may also be the fifth executive. Each of these executives has the right to vote at the board; other senior managers may sit as non-voting members.

The trust will then have a group which oversees its strategic and operational management. This would be the executives joined by other senior managers in the trust. Size and membership of this group will vary between trusts; often there will be clinical representation beyond the nursing and medical directors. *A Spoonful of Sugar* recommends that the chief pharmacist should have influence at this level; chief pharmacists are more likely to be included if they head a directorate or division, perhaps representing other non-medical groups [10].

The trust will then be organised into a number of manageable groups, typically divisions or directorates or care groups. Divisions group together a range of services led by a management team or general manager. An example of a division would be surgical specialities, which could include general surgery, orthopaedics, ophthalmology and gynaecology. In larger trusts a division may include up to 1000 staff and have a budget of tens of millions, with a drug spend of several millions. A directorate or care group structure would be along similar lines but the name suggests a larger number of smaller groupings. Orthopaedics, child health and general medicine could each form its own directorate. Figure 1.1 shows the directorate structure for Southampton University Hospitals NHS trust in 2002.

The management groupings of the organisation (directorate or division) would typically have a mixture of general, financial and clinical management input. Usually a senior nurse as well as a doctor would be part of the management team. Information officers would also support the business of the directorate or division.

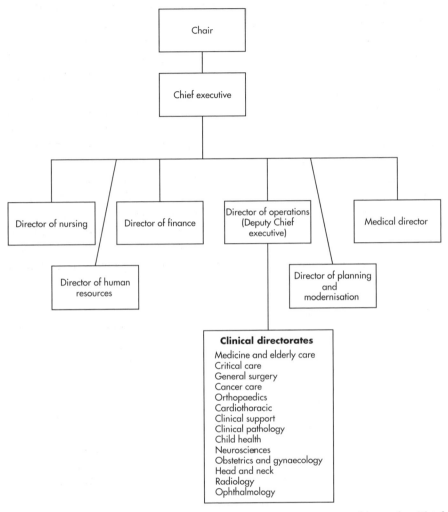

Figure 1.1 An example of a trust structure: executives accountable to the Chief Executive and details of clinical directorates.

Pharmacy's place in a trust

The move to involve doctors in management of trusts in the 1990s often left pharmacy as a loose end. No one structure has emerged as the way in which pharmacy should fit into a hospital's structure. In a directorate structure a large pharmacy service could stand alone, headed by the chief pharmacist, although the size of budget, even in larger departments (£2–3 million, excluding drugs), would be small for a typical directorate. Combining with other non-medical-led services such as physiotherapy or dietetics has been a path followed in a number of trusts. Chief pharmacists may act as lead or general manager for these groupings. Another model is where a general manager, possibly at executive level, has responsibility for a range of services that includes pharmacy. Grouping pharmacy with other non-bedholding specialities such as pathology, theatres and radiology in clinical support divisions is also possible. Whatever the structure, it is important that the chief pharmacist has responsibility for the service and the way in which medicines are used in the trust, having access to the executive when necessary.

The development of clinical pharmacy has led to staff specialising in various clinical areas. There are examples of pharmacists moving from a central pharmacy service to individual clinical directorates or divisions. This can increase the ability and opportunity of working with the multidisciplinary team and for specialists to feel ownership for their pharmacy service. However, it could lead to a

Table 1.3   Pharmacy staffing groups

Job title	Qualifications
Pharmacists	Members of the pharmaceutical society (UK or Northern Ireland)
Technicians	Qualified staff, having BTEC or NVQ (level 3) or an earlier equivalent in pharmaceutical science. Employed as medical technical officers (MTOs)
Assistants	Not formally qualified in pharmaceutical science but usually undergoing relevant competency or in-house training to undertake practical tasks in pharmacy. May be employed as assistant technical officers (ATOs) or on ancillary or local grades. NVQ (level 2) in development
Clerical and administrative staff	Undertaking personal assistant, administrative roles at senior level or in supportive capacity. May have considerable experience and relevant qualifications or be undertaking training
Other staff	Graduates from science or other backgrounds may take on roles within the service, for example, in quality control laboratories. Roles in storekeeping or purchasing or information technology may also bring in experienced or non-pharmaceutically qualified staff

NVQ, National Vocational Qualification.

more fragmented service or leave an isolated rump service of the non-devolved part of pharmacy.

Pharmacy needs to be involved not just in the management structure of the trust but in the wide variety of committees and groups within the trust. Once again, these vary between trusts but will include groups that deal with clinical governance, risk management, patient

Table 1.4 Pharmacists' grades and roles

Grade	Role
Basic-grade pharmacists (grades A/B)	Typically these are training grades organised on a rotational basis for the first few years after qualification. Experience is gained across the range of pharmaceutical specialities and is usually accompanied by further training and development: diploma or other qualification in clinical or similar subject. Competency-based training is being developed
Middle-grade pharmacists (I) (grade C)	Sometimes progression to C-grade is automatic, a part of the development programme for junior staff. Training may continue to be a large part of the role, with rotation through specialities continuing. However, specific responsibilities may be taken on or work may be fixed in one clinical speciality
Middle-grade pharmacists (II) (grade D)	Seen as the career grade for many staff. Around 36% of all posts in England and Wales in 2001 were at this grade [12]. More responsibility is carried than at C-grade, or having a specialised role. Typical grading for clinical pharmacists looking after a particular speciality
More senior-grade pharmacists (grades E/F)	These more senior staff have gained a reasonable level of experience and have either taken on a management or a specialist role. Running a large medicines information centre at district level, responsibility for a clinical service in a district general hospital or working as a specialist directorate pharmacist in a large teaching trust may be at these grades
Top grades (grades F/G/H)	Chief pharmacists would be graded at these levels or at a similar level on a management scale. Specialist pharmacists running a service at a regional centre or across a regional patch would also be graded at this level. Exceptionally, other specialist posts may be at this level

liaison, clinical effectiveness/audit, control of infection, health and safety and medicines. Pharmacy managers and staff need to create informal networks and contacts within the trust to ensure that as issues relating to medicines arise, appropriate advice and support are sought. Such contacts are just as important as the formal trust structures.

Pharmacy staff

Hospital pharmacy has developed a range of support staff roles. The introduction to this book mentioned several documents that encouraged the development of the technician role: the training and development of technicians have been crucial in the progress hospital pharmacy has made in clinical and medicines management services. Ensuring other support staff underpin and allow good use of resources is also important for pharmacy. The roles and job titles seen in pharmacy at the time of writing are shown in Tables 1.3–1.5.

Trusts have had the ability to develop local terms and conditions to deal with local needs, but the pattern is similar. Pay modernisation is

Table 1.5 Technician grades

Grade	Role and duties
Technicians (MTO 1 and 2)	Undertaking technical duties such as dispensing, aseptic preparation and roles such as checking, medication management at ward level and other patient-focused roles. Extended roles may be recognised with enhanced gradings
Senior technicians (MTO 3)	Typically, managing the technical work of a section of pharmacy, supervising other staff. Roles such as training NVQ students may be graded at this level
Management grades (MTO 4 and 5)	Undertaking the management of an area (dispensary or aseptic services, for example) or for a service across the pharmacy department. The highest grade is reserved for the most demanding, complex or autonomous posts

MTO, medical technical officer, NVQ, National Vocational Qualification.

part of revising the NHS: *Agenda for Change* will see changes in pay structures and impact on career structures [11].

Progression through the current (or future) grades follows a variety of routes. Aspirations and career pathways do not follow a simple pattern, however Table 1.6 gives a few examples of career histories based on current senior pharmacists.

The future

The NHS plan has laid out the key features of a reformed NHS. New technologies and changes in demographics and expectations will continue to impact on the service. Significant investment from general taxation is promised to support the reforms. The structure of the NHS is likely to evolve; further PCT mergers may take place; acute trusts may seek to move services out to primary and social care, leaving them as

Table 1.6   Examples of career pathways for hospital pharmacists

Case A
Hospital preregistration year (multisite)
Basic-grade pharmacist at a district general hospital (DGH): 1 year
Basic grade with role in peripheral hospitals: 18 months
Medicines information and clinical pharmacist (DGH): 3 years
Elderly care and education lead at teaching hospital: 18 months
Dispensary and clinical services manager at small teaching hospital: 16 months
Chief pharmacist at DGH: 8 years
Chief pharmacist and clinical director large teaching trust

Case B
Bradford undergraduate and preregistration
Junior rotational pharmacist (DGH): 3 years
Grade C in medicines information (DGH): 1 year
Medicines information pharmacist in drug industry: 4 years
Senior medicines information pharmacist (DGH): 1 year
Senior medicines information pharmacist in regional centre (deputy to regional lead)

Case C
Preregistration year in teaching hospital
Rotational junior pharmacist post (DGH): 2 years
Clinical pharmacist at teaching hospital: 18 months
Directorate pharmacist for surgery (DGH): 18 months
Directorate pharmacist for surgery (job-share) (DGH): 3 years
Principal clinical pharmacist (not full-time) (DGH)

high-tech, short-stay centres, supported by one-stop diagnostic and treatment units. The concept of foundation hospitals – trusts with greater independence – will also have an impact on the NHS landscape. It is clear from *A Spoonful of Sugar* [10] and from the obvious pressures on drug budgets that pharmacy has an important role to play in the future NHS – contributing to patient care, reducing the risks of medicines use and helping to achieve financial balance.

References

1. Department of Health. *The NHS Plan*. London: The Stationery Office, 2000.
2. Department of Health. *Shifting the Balance of Power Within the NHS: Securing Delivery*. London: The Stationery Office, 2001.
3. Hall N, chair. *Report of the Working Party Investigating the Hospital Pharmaceutical Service*. London: HMSO, 1970.
4. Griffiths Report. *NHS Management Enquiry*. London: HMSO, 1983.
5. Department of Health. *The New NHS: Modern, Dependable*. London: The Stationery Office, 1997.
6. Department of Health. *A First Class Service, Quality in the New NHS*. London: The Stationery Office, 1998.
7. Department of Health. *Our Healthier Nation*. London: The Stationery Office, 1999.
8. Department of Health. *Shifting the Balance of Power Within the NHS: The Next Steps*. London: The Stationery Office, 2001.
9. Department of Health. *Pharmacy in the Future*. London: Department of Health, 2000.
10. Audit Commission. *A Spoonful of Sugar – Medicines Management in NHS Hospitals*. London: Audit Commission, 2001.
11. Department of Health. *Agenda for Change, Modernising the NHS Pay System*. London: Department of Health, 1999.
12. Anonymous. Too few trainees in hospital pharmacy. *Pharm J* 2002; 268: 599.

Further reading

Department of Health website (2002). www.doh.gov.uk (accessed 10 November 2002).

Hallett L. *HSJ Guide to What's Happening in the NHS?* London: emap Public Sector Management, 2000.

Klein R. *The New Politics of the National Health Service*, 4th edn. Harlow: Pearson Education, 2001.

NHS website (2002). www.nhs.uk (accessed 10 November 2002).

2

Purchasing medicines

Howard Stokoe and David Samways

This chapter describes how English National Health Service (NHS) hospitals contract for the supply of medicines and explains typical local arrangements for obtaining medicines, invoicing and stock management. Although approaches are reasonably consistent across the whole of the UK, readers should note that the home countries organise themselves in different ways and that systems vary across the whole of Europe.

Background

Expenditure

The pharmaceutical market in the UK forms the context for hospital purchasing. The UK represents around 3% of the global market for medicines. NHS UK hospital expenditure represents about a fifth of the NHS total for prescription medicines, with the balance being spent in primary care. In 2000–2001 this hospital segment of the market was worth more than £1.6 billion. This sum excludes VAT, but it should be noted that hospitals do pay VAT on medicines and this element is included within their expenditure figures – figures for general practitioner (GP) prescribing costs do not include VAT.

The Pharmaceutical Price Regulation Scheme (PPRS)

The PPRS is a UK government scheme that regulates the profits that pharmaceutical companies can make when selling branded prescription medicines to the NHS [1]. At the same time, the scheme supports an industry that will continue to offer innovative medicines and is competitive internationally. Indeed, the UK pharmaceutical industry is seen as a significant asset; *The NHS Plan* makes this clear and also states that there needs to be opportunity for companies to undertake research with reasonable haste [2].

Under the PPRS suppliers are allowed to introduce major new medicines (new active substances) to the NHS at prices that they determine but can only increase prices with the Department of Health's agreement. The PPRS distinguishes the UK market from all others in the European Union (EU).

Generic substitution

Unlike the system in primary care, NHS hospital pharmacies dispense medicines generically, irrespective of how they are prescribed. Thus a brand name may be used by the doctor but a generic version may be issued. Exceptions are made if the branded product has unique characteristics (modified release, for example) that could result in a clinically important effect if substituted.

Aims of the service

Obtaining drugs from manufacturers, wholesalers and short-line stores is, of course, an essential part of the pharmaceutical service. Purchasing needs to be carried out with probity and to be undertaken efficiently. There are also conflicting demands on the service – a need to avoid being unable to meet a patient's need whilst not retaining too high a stock within the pharmacy. Too large a stock holding means that trust money is tied up in an asset; high stock levels may also lead to waste and will require more space than would a reasonable stock level. The Value for Money Unit with the NHS Benchmarking Reference Centre included some targets on a range of purchasing matters in their good-practice guides [3]. They state that a stock turnover rate of 11–13 times a year is 'good practice', while 14–15 times a year is 'better practice' – this would mean that a pharmacy issuing £6 million of medicines each year would carry around £410 000 stock – less than 4 weeks' supply – if it is to achieve the highest standard.

History

The first hospital contracts

Regional pharmaceutical officers and supplies managers introduced some of the first hospital contracts for medicines during the 1970s in the days of the regional health authorities (RHAs). At that time, therefore, purchasing was organised on a regional basis (see chapter 1 for details of the NHS structure). As branded medicines came off patent, and generic versions were introduced, these contracts were awarded to reflect a fall in price, as well as the additional benefit of competition between generic suppliers. Given that hospital pharmacists were able to dispense generically, the contracts delivered immediate cash savings that were then available to support the funding of newer, relatively more expensive and innovative medicines.

The MMM report

In 1986 the Modern Materials Management (MMM) Consultancy Group published an independent report *Investigation into the Provision of Pharmaceuticals to Health Authorities* on behalf of the NHS [4]. This proposed that each RHA set up a store (so-called short-line) to handle low-volume/high-value lines. These stores continue to exist and provide an option for the distribution of contract lines.

The impact of NHS reorganisations

In 1996, the RHAs and their associated management structures were disbanded. Even so, the regional drug contracting committees, that had been part of the old RHA arrangements, decided to continue, elected their own chair and continued operating as purchasing groups, using NHS Supplies to manage their contracts.

Subsequently NHS Supplies was reorganised to create a national supplies body that was in turn to become the Purchasing and Supply Agency (PaSA) during 2002.

Boundary changes and questions of performance

These and other issues, particularly the imposed changes to the boundaries of some purchasing groups, stimulated a demand by some pharmacists for an independent review of contracting performance. As a result, the Unit for Health Services Development consulted widely about the pros and cons of the contracting arrangements and what could be done to improve them. The resulting report, *A Generic Perspective*, represented probably the first meaningful attempt to describe the contracting arrangements in any depth and provided a common agenda for the purchasing groups, the pharmaceutical industry and the then NHS

Supplies 'to get it right' [5]. The recommendations of the report are now being implemented.

Overlaid on this background and history has been the impact of EU legislation.

Hospital procurement and the application of EU legislation

Background and requirements

The UK is a member state of the EU and an aim of the EU is to create a single European market devoid of all trading restrictions and barriers – a market place in which all businesses have an equal opportunity to compete. The EU regulates and monitors all large-scale public sector procurement through EU directives covering the supply of goods, services and works. In the UK the directives apply to all NHS contracting authorities, including health authorities and NHS trusts.

As a result of EU membership, hospital procurement is subject to the directives within the Treaty of Rome, including Article 12 (prohibition of discrimination on grounds of nationality), Article 28 (free movement of goods within the EU), and Article 81 (prohibition of agreements that prevent, restrict or distort competition).

The main requirements are:

- the advertisement of large public contracts to a standard format in the supplement to the *Official Journal of the European Community* (OJEC) so that suitable suppliers from all EU and government procurement agreement (GPA) countries have the opportunity to declare their interest
- prescribed minimum periods for responses
- the use of technical specifications which are non-discriminatory and which refer to EU or other recognised international standards wherever possible
- the use of objective criteria for selecting participants and awarding contracts.

The directives only apply where the value of the procurement exceeds a given threshold. This is quoted in euros (a contract value of £90 000 will generally serve as a 'rule of thumb').

Types of procedure

The regulations recognise three contracting procedures:

- An **open procedure** that is available in all circumstances and involves only a single stage. All offers received must be considered, provided that candidates have passed any minimum shortlisting criteria. The open procedure can be conducted more quickly than the restricted procedure but there is no possibility of limiting the number of bids received.

- A **restricted procedure** that is also available in all circumstances but involves a two-stage procedure. From amongst the candidates expressing interest (the first stage) it is then possible to shortlist a limited number from whom to invite offers (the second stage).

- A **negotiated procedure** is the most flexible but the least transparent of the three procedures. It is used only in very limited circumstances (for example, where goods are needed extremely urgently due to reasons that were unforeseeable by, and not attributable to, the buyer).

Offer evaluation

The directives require that the contract must be awarded to the candidate who submits the lowest-priced tender or the tender which is the most economically advantageous (buyers almost invariably select the latter because it gives them greater flexibility). The factors that may be used to determine economic advantage include price, quality of service and running costs: the chosen factors must be stated in the OJEC notice or the contract documents.

Negotiation within the process

Where the open or restricted procedures are being used, the rules forbid buyers to engage in post-tender negotiations with candidates. These are defined as negotiations with candidates on fundamental aspects of their bids, for example, price. Discussions aimed as clarifying or supplementing the content of the bids are, on the other hand, permitted, provided all candidates are treated equally.

Pre-tender discussions with potential suppliers, conducted on an equitable basis, are critical to designing contracts that will perform and deliver.

Types of contract

There are two types of contract:

- The **commitment contract** commits a legal entity (such as an NHS trust) to purchase a defined quantity of product at a defined price.

- The **framework contract** does not guarantee to deliver commitment. Rather, based on estimated volumes, it provides (for example, on behalf of a group of hospitals represented as a purchasing group) a framework against which purchase orders will be placed by hospitals covered by the agreement.

The framework agreement sets the terms and conditions of the purchase by the hospital, including price/pricing schedule, with the true contract being formed when individual hospitals place a purchase order.

Framework contracts are normally used on behalf of purchasing groups in recognition that an agent (such as PaSA) or a hospital within the purchasing group cannot deliver absolute commitment to volume on behalf of the group.

The strengths of the contracting process

It may appear sometimes that the contracting process is cumbersome and bureaucratic. However, recognition must be paid to its inherent strengths. These are that the process is auditable, is legal (so minimises the risk of challenge, particularly where the lowest bid is not accepted), utilises sealed-bid tenders, is based on a set of stages and rules that provide a framework for equal treatment for all bidders, establishes a clear trading basis between the NHS and its suppliers (through standard terms and conditions) and provides a fair test of value for money on behalf of the NHS.

The organisation of hospital contracts

Hospitals have contracts at various levels. These levels are local (trust), purchasing group and, very rarely, national.

The principles of purchasing group contracts are straightforward. Hospitals aggregate their purchasing power through their pharmacy purchasing groups and the PaSA then competitively tenders, awards and manages the resulting contracts, as an agent, on behalf of the groups. Each trust must nominate an individual to represent the interests of its hospital managers, clinicians and budget-holders (as well as its local relationships with primary care trusts) on its purchasing group. The nominee's roles include sharing information, adjudicating contracts and participating in collective dialogue with the PaSA buyer dedicated to work with the group.

The nominees use their knowledge and experience that originate in managing medicines on a day-to-day basis (particularly through formulary management systems that are linked to drugs and therapeutics committees, and input into the prescribing process) to direct the management of contracts.

In England there are six main purchasing groups operating on a geographical basis with some, varying by main group, being divided into smaller groups and purchasing consortia. Each main group 'owns' a contract of between 1500 and 2000 lines, representing upward of 200 suppliers. Whilst the contracts on behalf of these groups are framework contracts that do not guarantee commitment, the ownership of the contracts (through the participation of their member trusts) ensures that these contracts are highly effective.

Framework contracts on behalf of each purchasing group last for a period of 2 years and include options to extend for an additional 2 years, and for a further 2 years on top of this (this is described as the 2 + 2 + 2 model), if this is required. With this contracting model a main group contract will be tendered on behalf of a purchasing group once within any 2-year period and with a 4-month period between each contract being tendered. This allows the experience gained from letting one contract to be translated into the next tender (a mutual benefit for both the NHS and its suppliers). Figure 2.1 illustrates the contracting cycle.

The 'overlapping' approach is intended to enable purchasing groups to focus on award decisions that require dedication of time and effort, for example, where there are significant clinical or strategic issues to consider. This approach allows additional contracts to be let, on behalf of a purchasing group, at any time. When this is undertaken it is usually with the objective of ultimate incorporation into the main contract.

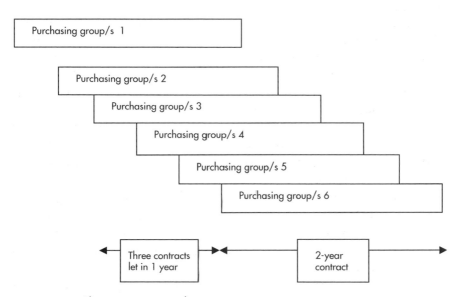

Figure 2.1 The contracting cycle.

The main purchasing groups tend to focus on contract awards for true generics (where the award reflects collective purchasing decisions) rather than those that reflect clinical commitment (for example, therapeutic selection) where, the belief is, this is best delivered through smaller groups.

Systems and processes

Pharmacy specialists and working relationships with PaSA

Technical and procurement specialists within pharmacy strengthen the contracting arrangements, especially where they are employed by a trust to support and work with a purchasing group. Pharmacy quality control (QC) arrangements are involved in assessing product quality as part of the tendering process, as well as on a day-to-day basis (see chapter 5 for further detail on QC services).

Specialist involvement, combined with the day-to-day working relationships between the trusts and their PaSA buyer, minimises duplication of effort through shared access to central contract management and associated procurement expertise.

PaSA management systems

PaSA manages the contracting process using a single management system – pharmacy tendering evaluation (PHATE). PHATE maintains a database of all suppliers and product lines. It generates invitations to tender (through an electronic format) and produces comparative evaluations to support contract adjudication before finally generating award notices to suppliers and contract details to trusts (currently in both paper and electronic formats).

Meeting structures

The totality of the contracting arrangements is underpinned through meeting arrangements and communication structures. The pharmacy purchasing groups, elected chair and their PaSA buyers meet regularly to share information, adjudicate contracts and monitor performance. Representatives of the purchasing groups (two from each division) meet every 3 months with PaSA representatives at the National Pharmaceutical Supplies Group (NPSG), along with a Department of Health observer, to set general strategic direction.

Recent changes

Parallel imports

The free movement of goods within the EU has opened up the hospital contracts to include parallel-imported and parallel-distributed medicines. Hospitals have used these to gain additional discounts, although these gains may only be short-lived as the UK price may also fall.

Issues to watch

Both the NHS and supplier environments continue to change, ensuring that the market remains highly dynamic. Particular issues to be aware of include the impact of:

- the Competition Act following the Office of Fair Trading ruling on Napp Pharmaceuticals
- EU rulings concerning the free movement of goods
- price harmonisation trends within the EU
- the fact that the current PPRS will run until at least 2004 subject to a midterm review, which either the Department of Health or the Association of the British Pharmaceutical Industry may request from 1 April 2002
- the increasing influence of commissioners on hospital contracting arrangements
- the ongoing changes within the regulatory environment; company mergers and their impact on the pharmaceutical supply chain
- the impact of e-commerce and the introduction of consistent NHS systems.

Local arrangements

The majority of pharmacy departments now use information technology systems for ordering, goods receipt and invoice processing. These systems are configured so that the audit requirement for segregation of these tasks between different staff members is delivered. Procedures must be consistent with the trust's standing financial instructions. Manual systems are very occasionally used but these will be phased out and will not be covered here.

Ordering

Items which need to be ordered will be identified by the computer system or by pharmacy staff. Computer systems maintain live stock levels and as these fall to the reorder level, the item is flagged for reorder. The reorder level is either fixed or can be calculated by the system based on an algorithm of average daily usage, time it takes to be delivered (lead time) and a preset safety factor. Infrequently used items may be flagged so that they are only placed on order by authorised staff.

The system will allocate these items to a preferred supplier which will be:

- the contract holder
- the manufacturer offering an NHS hospital price
- a short-line store
- a wholesaler.

These lists of items will be reviewed and amended by an authorised member of staff and orders generated. The supplier may be changed if the lead time is not appropriate for patient needs or the preferred supplier is out of stock. The orders will be sent to the supplier by one of the following methods.

- Verbally by phone: this method is useful if the item is very urgent or is patient-specific. If used routinely, verbal ordering is very labour-intensive and subject to transcription errors.
- Faxing: this reduces transcription errors but requires re-entering of data by the supplier and is dependent on the quality of the faxed copy.
- Electronic data interchange (EDI): this is the exchange of electronic order data. It is the objective for all NHS ordering. The accuracy is dependent on the upkeep of product codes and so on, but it has the potential for rapid, accurate transfer, with minimal time commitment for staff.
- Post: this route is now rarely used due to time delay and cost.

Goods receipt

On receipt, goods will be checked visually for damage and expiry date. They will then be checked against the delivery note and against either a hard copy or computer copy of the order. The aim is to ensure that quantities and products are correct and that there are no obvious defects – that there are no damaged goods. Any discrepancies will be notified to the supplier immediately. Many trusts collect data on errors and timeliness of deliveries since supplier performance is a key consideration at contract adjudication. Once checks are complete, items will be entered into the computer system and stock levels updated.

Batch number details are recorded in some trusts although the benefit of this is reduced by the inability to track batches to the end-user. There is a requirement to do this with blood products.

When controlled drugs are ordered and receipted, the requirements of the Misuse of Drugs regulations must be followed. Records of receipt are made in a register and the balance of stock record updated.

Invoicing

Practice varies between trusts: this function is carried out by pharmacy staff in approximately 80% of trusts and by finance department staff in the remainder. Wherever it is carried out, the system requires input of invoice data into the computer system and checking of price invoiced against price expected on original order. Most trusts require exact matching of contract line prices and agreed tolerances with non-contract lines. This is because most systems do not routinely update non-contract prices but use last purchase price on the orders.

Historically, invoices have been received in hard copy with details manually entered into the computer system. The receipt of electronic invoice files and subsequent matching of items is developing rapidly and is used to some extent in 20% of trusts. These systems automatically process items with complete matching of data and allow trust staff to focus on price or delivery discrepancies.

Acceptance of the invoice details will update the unit cost of the item(s) on the computer system and also authorise payment to the supplier.

The future

The introduction of integrated electronic patient record systems across the NHS and the development of web-based e-commerce packages will radically change the procurement of pharmaceuticals. This will change the role of pharmacy staff from being process-focused to a more strategic role supporting clinical objectives of the trust. The Audit Commission has indicated the need for trusts to make best use of supplies expertise and contract purchasing [6]. The demand to achieve effective and efficient purchasing for hospital medicines will continue. The National Purchasing and Supply Agency (NPSA) has summarised the recommendations to develop such services in its *Review of NHS Pharmaceutical Contracting* [7]. The procurement role will continue to form a building block for effective hospital pharmacy services.

References

1. ABPI. *Understanding the PPRS*. London: ABPI, 1999.
2. Department of Health. *The NHS Plan*. London: The Stationery Office, 2000.

3.   Value for Money Unit and the NHS Benchmarking Reference Centre. *Pharmacy Good Practice Guides*. Wrexham: NHS Wales, 1996.

4.   MMM Consultancy Group. *Investigation into the Provision of Pharmaceuticals to Health Authorities*. MMM: 1986.

5.   Mounsey C, Curtis S A. *A Generic Perspective*. London: The Unit for Health Service Development, 1988.

6.   Audit Commission. *A Spoonful of Sugar – Medicines Management in NHS Hospitals*. London: Audit Commission, 2001.

7.   NPSA. *NHS Hospital Pharmaceutical Services, Review of NHS Pharmaceutical Contracting*. Reading: NPSA, 2002.

Further reading

Farley P. Purchasing pharmaceuticals – obtaining the most pills for the pound. *Pharm Management* 1996; 12: 50–52.

Guild of Healthcare Pharmacists procurement special interest group website. www.ghp.org.uk/default.asp?channel_id+394&editorial_id=8587 (accessed 12 November 2002).

Mounsey C, Curtis S A. *A Generic Perspective*. London: The Unit for Health Service Development, 1988.

NPSA. *NHS Hospital Pharmaceutical Services, Review of NHS Pharmaceutical Contracting*. Reading: NPSA, 2002.

Samways D, Wind K, Page J. Towards 'intelligent' purchasing. *Hosp Pharm* 2001; 8: 144–146.

Scrip is a journal issued twice a week by PJB Publications. See website at www.pjbpubs.com (accessed 12 November 2002).

Stokoe H. Pharmacy procurement: generics contracting in England. *Hosp Pharm* 2000; 7: 42–44.

3

Medicines supply

John W Barnett

Supply of medicines is part of a multidisciplinary process, triggered by the writing of a prescription and ending with administration, which is necessary for the treatment of nearly all patients. The safe and secure handling of medicines is an essential part of a trust's medicines management system and is the subject of one of the standards in the Department of Health controls assurance framework (see chapter 9), which seeks to manage risk. Medicines supply, as with other aspects of such systems, should be undertaken within a framework of policies, procedures, staff training and quality assurance measures.

A key requirement is that responsibilities for each component are clearly defined, normally in the trust's medicines policy. The Controls Assurance Standard for Medicines Management gives guidance in Criterion 1 that, whilst the Chief Executive has the overall statutory responsibility, the Chief Pharmacist 'should be responsible for ensuring that systems are in place to appropriately address all aspects of the safe and secure handling of medicines and report directly to the Chief Executive for this purpose across the whole of the organisation' [1]. This re-emphasizes the role of the 'Senior Pharmacist' described in the Duthie Report, which also gives guidance on the responsibilities of other professionals in the handling of medicines [2].

The multidisciplinary nature of the processes involved means that they are more prone to error, for example through communication failures, than would be the case with a relatively complex process undertaken by a single profession. It is important to ensure that there is a team approach and that the different insights of medical and nursing colleagues are sought on existing processes and any proposed changes. Joint action will be needed to achieve the Department of Health target of a reduction of serious medication errors by 40% by 2005.

Systems of supply should be chosen to minimise the potential for medication errors. Security measures should minimise the risk of misappropriation of medicines by staff, to protect them and the wider community. Chosen methods should also:

- allow efficient utilisation of hospital personnel
- control costs, including minimising wastage
- ensure timely provision of the medicine
- meet legislative, professional and any particular local or patient group requirements.

History

A milestone in the adoption of security measures into medicine supply occurred with the publication of the Aitken Report in 1958, which recommended practices that are still followed today [3]. However, the key driver in the development of systems has been the desire to minimise medication errors. These were recognised as a major cause for concern during the 1960s and resulted in the introduction of new prescribing and administration recording systems, which form the basis for those in current use. The review of all prescriptions by a pharmacist was regarded as essential to new systems being developed. This never occurred for ward stock items, which are issued without reference to a prescription, and in Scotland all medicines were issued in this way. However, prescription sheets must not leave the ward, as other types of error can occur when they are not readily available. Pharmacists therefore began visiting the wards to see the prescription sheets – the start of today's clinical pharmacy.

Errors were known to occur more often when the nurse had to make selections from a wide range of drug or patient names. Introduction of a ward medicine trolley obviated the need for selection from the stock cupboard for each round. Early ward pharmacists either made the selection of drugs for the trolley or transcribed details to enable individual dispensing in the pharmacy [4, 5]. For systems using individually dispensed medicines, a trolley drawer for each patient again minimised selection error. Such trends led to unit dose systems and the use of patient bedside medicine cabinets in current practice also has the benefit of reducing selection error.

Current practice

Supply to inpatients

Storage arrangements

Responsibilities Ward storage of medicines, in almost all instances, will be in locked cupboards or another secure receptacle, e.g. a patient's medicines cabinet. The appointed nurse in charge, i.e. the registered nurse with continuing responsibility for the ward, or other profession-ally qualified person or nurse in charge of other clinical areas, must ensure that systems for the security of medicines are followed and that stocks are safeguarded [2]. He/she may delegate some of the duties, such as access, to another nurse or to a member of the pharmacy staff, but the responsibility always remains with him/her. The pharmaceutical service may assume responsibility for replenishment of these stocks, advise on the type and location of cupboards, regularly inspect and audit them and assure the quality of the product at the time of use. However, phar-macy staff are rarely in a position to do more than this as they do not administer or use the items stored.

Keys The keys to cupboards should be labelled, kept separate and carried on the person of a nurse (or other qualified person in charge). Controlled drug (CD) cupboard keys should be kept on a separate ring that can be readily identified and carried by the assigned nurse in charge, i.e. the senior registered nurse on duty for the ward or clinical area, iden-tified as nurse in charge for that shift. This all has the effect of minimis-ing unnecessary access to medicines. Secure arrangements are necessary for duplicate sets of keys and for those for areas that are not continu-ously staffed, with recording of signatures for them. For self-adminis-tration schemes patients may hold the key to their medicine cabinet and a master key is kept by the appointed nurse in charge.

Cupboards and trolleys Separate lockable cupboards should be avail-able for internal and external medicines (constructed to the British Standard specification) and CDs (see separate section in this chapter) [2]. In small units, if space does not permit a separate cupboard for external medicines, they must be kept on a separate shelf, below those for internal use. A separate lockable medicine refrigerator must be available in all areas where medicines may require it, with a maximum/minimum thermometer to enable at least weekly checks that temperatures are maintained in the range 2–8°C.

Medicines in current use on wards are either kept in a lockable trolley or in individual patient medicine cabinets or drawers, usually at the bedside; none of these must be used for permanent storage. The trolley must be immobilised when not in use, locked either in a cupboard or to a wall; it is not normally used for CDs. The patient medicine cabinets or drawers must be lockable and not readily portable [2].

Exceptions   Medicines not usually locked away are:

- medicines in emergency kits, in clearly labelled boxes with a tamper-evident seal, kept readily accessible
- intravenous fluids, antiseptics and irrigation solutions
- medicines considered appropriate for some patients to administer under the supervision of a registered nurse, unless there is a hazard to other patients.

This last situation is distinct from participation in a formally recognised self-administration scheme, which allows greater independence of action for patients and no limit on the range of medicines covered. The medicine is likely to be in one of the following categories:

- inhalers
- glyceryl trinitrate sublingual tablets or spray
- oral contraceptives and hormone replacement therapy products
- ointments or creams
- insulin preparations.

There must be a valid prescription for the medicine. The prescriber may specify that the patient should have ready access to the preparation (inhalers or glyceryl trinitrate), otherwise it is the registered nurse's decision (which should be documented) on whether to have the medicine on the patient's bedside locker. The patient must be capable of administering the medicine correctly and willing and able to tell the nurse when a dose has been taken so that this can be recorded on the prescription sheet.

Ordering ward stock

Nurse requisitioning   Safety and security are key issues here. Ward staff tend to accept that what is supplied by pharmacy is correct, even though the supply may be based on an ambiguous or poorly written requisition and without sight of the prescription. Procedures and documentation need to minimise opportunities for misappropriation and misunderstanding, for example if a medicine is ordered by telephone, could it be diverted, on receipt, without detection or an incorrect product supplied?

A minimum requirement to give an audit trail in a manual system is that the requisition has the signature of the ordering nurse, which pharmacy can verify, the issuer's signature is entered and a receipt is obtained. Serial numbering and book-fast copies (kept for a minimum of 2 years) minimise the opportunity for destruction of records to go undetected. Where requisition books are used there should be only one in each ward or department, kept locked away, with new ones treated as controlled stationery, stocked only in pharmacy [2].

Topping up   Responsibility for routine ordering of ward stock is transferred, under this system, from nursing staff to pharmacy technicians or assistants, who check and replenish this to predetermined levels, usually weekly. The requirements are either entered on a computer-printed copy of the ward stock list, perhaps able to be used over several weeks to show trends and in a sequence convenient for distribution staff, or input to hand-held terminals reading bar codes. The stock list should be based on usage and agreed between the appointed nurse and a designated member of pharmacy staff, usually a technician. Supplies are usually dispatched to the ward, in locked boxes, for nursing staff to store. A record of what has been supplied is kept on the ward and in the pharmacy, the latter including the signature of the nurse receiving the medicines.

This system allows much greater pharmacy control over the quality and quantity of medicines stored on the ward. It saves nursing time but is of major benefit to pharmacy in allowing a large block of work to be undertaken when pressures are least.

Individual patient supply

Non-stock dispensing   The choice of inpatient supply system for a hospital lies anywhere on a spectrum between total stock and almost complete individual dispensing. Whilst the former was the traditional Scottish system and the latter is favoured in private hospitals because it facilitates charging, the choice in National Health Service (NHS) hospitals throughout the UK should now be based on a careful risk appraisal of the options and resources (principally staff) available. Reasons for individual dispensing may include minimising the risk that the wrong patient receives a particularly unusual or toxic drug, the guarantee that the prescription must be seen by pharmacy, or control of non-formulary supplies. It may be used to promote return to pharmacy of unused, less common medicines when the patient is discharged. Labels do not normally include directions for use.

One-stop dispensing The concept is to combine inpatient and discharge dispensing into a single supply, labelled with directions for use. Manufacturers' original packs are usually dispensed and the patient is discharged with what remains after use in hospital. If this is less than a minimum quantity agreed with local general practitioners (GPs), usually 2 weeks' supply, an additional pack is issued. Large numbers of individually dispensed items cannot be handled in a conventional medicines trolley, so each patient normally has a bedside medicines cabinet, which can also be used for the patient's own drugs (see below) or in a self-administration scheme. These also reduce the risk of medication error by limiting the choices for selection at administration times and allow nurses to give more individualised patient care. There is a need to keep the contents of cabinets up-to-date with prescription changes and, at discharge, to check that the pack quantity and label are still appropriate and that the cabinet is empty, all of which may be done by a pharmacist or technician.

Funding has to be transferred to the trust from primary care for the extra days' supply of discharge medication, for any staff increases and for additional computer software, which may be needed to undertake costing to each GP practice in the scheme. However, because the Hospital Service is usually able to negotiate advantageous prices, there may well be an overall saving to the local health economy. Patients benefit by having patient information leaflets (PILs) provided (a statutory requirement), by avoiding the wait for discharge medicines to be dispensed, provided that the prescription is written in good time, and also by having more time before ordering repeat prescriptions. The hospital can meet its legal obligation on PILs and also benefits from speedier discharges.

The Royal Pharmaceutical Society's Hospital Pharmacists Group has produced useful guidance on the introduction of one-stop dispensing, use of patients' own drugs (PODs) and self-administration schemes [6]. Using patient packs at the time of discharge, a possible intermediate step to one-stop dispensing, has also been successful [7].

Patients' own drugs Patients admitted to hospital are usually asked to bring their medicines with them to facilitate the recording of their drug history. These were routinely returned to pharmacy for destruction once a hospital supply was obtained. However, the move to dispensing of prescriptions in primary care using manufacturers' original packs has given much greater confidence in their continued usefulness, but *only* for the patient to whom they were originally supplied.

In many hospitals PODs are routinely returned to the patient's home, as soon as possible after admission, with a relative or carer, with varying input as to whether the medicines are suitable for use. The medicines are legally the patient's property and handing them back simplifies hospital procedures and reduces the risk of failure to return them later, if appropriate. However, the patient, once discharged, may be confused as to whether previous medication should still be taken, perhaps because discharge medicines, although the same as before, have been labelled with different drug names, possibly leading to double-dosing. Alternatively, the treatment may have been changed, perhaps because it was the cause of admission, but risk remains while the previous medicines are in the home. This system places significant responsibility on the GP, as well as the nurse counselling the patient on discharge medicines, to explain which of the medicines at home should still be taken. The hospital may require some form of disclaimer to be signed when the medicines are handed back, because of these risks.

An alternative strategy is for patients' medicines, with their permission, to be sent to the hospital pharmacy, in a bag labelled with the patient's name, registration number, ward and number of containers, for either reissue (if appropriate) or destruction when the discharge prescription is dispensed. A problem with this process, which may arise particularly on surgical wards, is that the doctor may not prescribe a patient's continuing, long-term treatment on discharge, assuming the GP does not need to be informed and the patient has supplies at home. Delays occur while this is corrected to legitimise the return of the medicine to the patient. The hospital's computerised patient administration system needs to be checked at intervals to identify those who have been discharged without a discharge prescription, or when the pharmacy was closed, or before the PODs reached the department. The patient and/or GP may feel aggrieved at such losses through the system and be unwilling to have medicines brought in on future occasions, with the disadvantages inherent in the first system. Patients may be asked to sign disclaimer forms if they are unwilling to have their medicines returned to pharmacy under this system, following an explanation of any risks.

A major advantage of having a medicine cabinet for each patient is that PODs are not 'lost in the system'. They can be used, where appropriate, during the hospital stay, supplemented by one-stop dispensed items, and the balance issued at discharge with patient counselling. Before use their suitability must be assessed, with this being variously undertaken by pharmacists, technicians, doctors or nurses at different hospitals. The value of the overall financial savings varies with the costing of this step and also the type of patient concerned. However, significant benefits in patient care have been achieved with, at the very least, no extra cost [8]. Criteria for acceptability also vary between hospitals. An example of minimum requirements is that the medicine must be:

- still required by the patient
- able to be positively identified, with no mixing with other products or strengths. The possibility of a dispensing error having occurred should be considered
- in date, as shown by the expiry date if present, otherwise dispensed within the previous 6 months. Ophthalmic preparations should only be used until a new supply is obtained
- correctly labelled with patient name, product name and strength, supplier's address and date of dispensing
- of only one type or brand. Mixed batches in the same container are not accepted.

When the directions are inappropriate, relabelling by pharmacy staff may be permissible. As with one-stop dispensing (see above), further checks on directions and quantities are required on discharge. The importance of these, including the check that the locker has been emptied, has been shown by reported errors [9], which also highlight the need for thorough training of those involved. Guidance on implementation [6] includes the need for publicity to encourage patients to bring in their medicines.

Unit dose systems   Unit dose systems have been adopted quite widely in North America and many European countries but have only been tried to a very limited extent in the UK. The concept is that pharmacy provides medicines to wards in single unit packages, either just prior to the time of administration or on a daily or (for long-stay) weekly basis, placing them in the patient's individually labelled drawer in a medicine cabinet, trolley or cassette. As far as possible doses of liquid medicines are packaged in individual containers and tablets and capsules are individually wrapped in foil or cellophane. Ideally, injections are drawn up into the syringe, reconstituted or diluted if necessary. Each package is fully labelled with its contents (but not necessarily the patient's name), allowing positive identification of the contents up to the time of administration, thus reducing the potential for error. The number of doses supplied is sufficient until the next visit.

The main advantage of these systems is the reduction in the potential for medication error. In a trial in Leeds, replacing a complete ward stock system, a 54% reduction in the rate of administration errors was found [10]. Nursing time was saved but, even if it could be released, it would have been insufficient to compensate for the additional pharmacy staff requirement.

Supply to outpatients

Three options are available – dispensing by the hospital pharmacy, dispensing by a community pharmacist of a hospital doctor's prescription on form FP10(HP), or referral of patients back to their GP for prescribing on form FP10. The difference between these forms is important from a financial perspective as the costs of supply on FP10(HP)s are recharged to the trust, whereas those from use of FP10s are set against primary care budgets.

The option of referring patients back to their GP for prescribing is dependent on the acceptability of transfer of clinical responsibility [11]. In Scotland the GP always retains this, the outpatient being referred to the hospital only for a consultation, so prescription on GP10 forms is the norm. In England and Wales such transfer of prescribing was often seen as 'cost-shifting' of expensive treatments from hospital budgets to primary care. This was unpopular with GPs, when they had insufficient information to manage the patient safely, since ultimate liability lies with the doctor who signs the prescription. These problems can be overcome with shared-care agreements between the consultant and the GP on continuing care, once the patient's condition is stable, under a protocol normally provided by the hospital. For some patients the GP may prefer to initiate long-term treatment with a drug from the practice formulary.

The principal advantages of dispensing for outpatients from hospital pharmacy departments are:

- immediate commencement of treatment
- supply of hospital-only medicines
- facility to supply clinical trial material
- convenience of the patient, which may be clinically important if the prescription might not otherwise be 'cashed'
- easy access to the prescriber when queries arise
- maintaining compliance with the hospital formulary.

Financial savings are also often quoted as a reason for hospital dispensing but need to be carefully evaluated. Hospitals pay VAT on medicines, whereas dispensing by community pharmacists is zero-rated and advantageous prices obtained through hospital contracts may be insufficient to counterbalance this difference. Discounts vary with different groups of products, so some clinics may be more economically supplied through the hospital, others via community pharmacies. Staffing costs are also important, particularly for a dedicated outpatient pharmacy, where underutilised staff can mean a cost per prescription much higher than the community pharmacist's dispensing fee. The most significant factors, however, may be the quantity prescribed and whether the formulary is being followed; prescribers' compliance on both is often dependent on the hospital pharmacist's ability to intervene. National guidance in England [11] is that a minimum of 14 days' treatment should be supplied if hospital prescribing for outpatients is undertaken, and 7 days' for those treated in accident and emergency (A&E). Supplies may be limited to these periods for hospital dispensing but exceeded on FP10(HP)s. However, as with discharge medicines, there is now a move to 28-day outpatient dispensing to realise the benefits of using manufacturers' original packs [12]. The FP10(HP) forms are eventually returned to the trust, after dispensing and pricing, but this may be too late to gain any benefit from feedback of audit results.

Dispensing by a hospital pharmacy may not necessarily mean direct contact with patients as medicines may be posted to them. Alternatively, suitably labelled prepacked medicines for standard treatments may be issued to departments (e.g. A&E) for medical or nursing staff to insert the patient's name; a register of issues is needed to maintain an audit trail and reduce the potential for abuse. Predictable requirements for day-case patients following surgery may be able to be dispensed in advance and issued after the pharmacy has closed.

A disadvantage to the patient of hospital dispensing can be the waiting time involved, although there may be scope for the pharmacy to take measures which produce a significant improvement [13]. A major disadvantage to the hospital is that it deflects pharmacists and technicians from a clinical role on the wards. In 1988 the Department of Health, in a health circular requiring health authorities to plan for implementation of clinical pharmacy [14], suggested that 'subject to a satisfactory local option-appraisal exercise' use of FP10(HP) forms could be used, 'thereby releasing hospital staff for other duties'. Outpatient dispensing by hospitals is further challenged in the Welsh *Report of the Task and Finish Group for Prescribing* [15], which recommends that this should only occur when there is an urgent clinical need and in the Audit Commission report [16], which in paragraph 64 suggests that 'the practice ... should be questioned'.

Controlled drugs in hospital

Handling of CDs in hospitals is subject to legislation, NHS guidance (Duthie and Aitkin Reports [2, 3]) and any additional local requirements specified in the trust's medicines policy. Some variation between hospitals is therefore inevitable. The following paragraphs are intended as a simplified guide on some aspects of where law and guidance meet. A useful fact sheet on legal aspects is available from the Royal Pharmaceutical Society's website (www.rpsgb.org.uk).

Prescriptions

Prescriptions are always required in hospital practice. They must meet the requirements of the *Misuse of Drugs Regulations 2001* [17] if they are dispensed in the pharmacy for an individual patient. Facsimile prescriptions cannot be accepted to facilitate the supply of a CD on a discharge prescription. No CD can be considered for inclusion in a patient group direction.

Ordering

Stocks of CDs for wards, operating theatres or other departments are obtained by the sister or acting sister in charge, using duplicate requisitions that are of standard design throughout the NHS (and usually also used in private hospitals) to meet legal requirements. Their signatures should be checked against a list provided by nurse management. Operating department practitioners are not yet legally authorised to requisition. Only one requisition book should be in use in each ward or department, kept locked away, and new ones should be treated as controlled stationery, stocked only in pharmacy [2]. All requisitions and copies must be kept for a minimum of 2 years.

Record keeping

Ward and theatre CD registers are required by NHS guidance, though not regulations, and, in the NHS, are of a standard design. Their use should be regarded as mandatory. The stock balance of CDs should be reconciled 'for good practice' at least once every 24 hours by two nurses, according to Duthie [2]. If a discrepancy does arise, this frequency minimises the number of nurses to be questioned. Registers should be kept for a minimum of 2 years from the date of the last entry.

Administration/supply

A second nurse should check all aspects of the administration of CDs according to Duthie [2], but there is no statutory requirement. The sister or acting sister (assigned nurse in charge) cannot supply a CD, other than for administration to a patient, and this has implications when a dose of a CD is required urgently from another ward. The administration must be recorded in the register of the ward from which the drug is taken, witnessed by a nurse from that ward. If such a practice is allowed in the hospital, it will be defined in the medicines policy.

Disposal

Expired stocks still on the ward are outside the scope of the regulations. Their destruction does not, therefore, need the attendance of an authorised person and can be witnessed by a nurse and pharmacist, if allowed by local policy, with entries in the register. Local arrangements must also be defined for disposal of partly used ampoules.

PODs can be destroyed in the pharmacy without the presence of an authorised person but here the record should be separate from the department's register. Special considerations apply to illegal substances taken from patients and a policy on this should be agreed with the hospital's legal adviser and included in the local medicines policy.

Storage

In private hospitals, CDs (Schedules 2 and 3, with some exceptions) in the pharmacy and on the wards must be stored in safes, cabinets or rooms which either comply with a detailed specification given in the *Misuse of Drugs (Safe Custody) Regulations 1973* [18] or have a police certificate to confirm they provide an adequate degree of security. The legal requirement for NHS hospitals is that the CDs are kept in a locked receptacle (no specification), only to be opened by a person who can lawfully be in possession, e.g. the sister or acting sister, or somebody acting on his/her behalf. The Duthie Report [2] is ambiguous on ward storage of CDs, stating 'For Controlled Drugs the Misuse of Drugs (Safe Custody) regulations apply', which could be interpreted as either continuation of the status quo or as recommending storage in cupboards meeting the detailed specification of the regulations. Many have adopted this latter course for cupboards purchased since 1988. The previous design, an inner cabinet for CDs (not to the standard of the regulations) within an outer cupboard fitted with a red warning light to show when it is unlocked, is still available to purchase, as well as continuing to be used in areas which have not been upgraded. For new CD storage arrangements in the pharmacy, it is often beneficial to have police advice, even though not legally required. CD cupboards should not, generally, be used for storage of anything else (including patient valuables) to minimise the occasions when access is required. However, it has been suggested that potassium chloride ampoules might be kept there to avoid inadvertent administration in place of sodium chloride [19]. CDs dispensed for individual patients in a self-administration scheme can be kept in their bedside medicines cabinet.

Clinical trials

A clinical trial is an investigation by a doctor or dentist involving administration of a medicinal product to a patient to assess the product's safety and efficacy (a Medicines Control Agency definition). The prescribing of an unlicensed product for an individual named patient does not automatically constitute a trial.

The pharmacist has a key role in the organisation and management of clinical trials, which is much wider than the supply function, and this is reflected in guidelines from the Royal Pharmaceutical Society. These guidelines suggest that one pharmacist should be designated to take special responsibility for clinical trials and describe, in some detail, suggested responsibilities for review of and advice on the protocol, setting up the trial, dispensing and ongoing administration. Medical Research Council guidelines endorse a 'suitably experienced' pharmacist's involvement in planning a trial.

All research studies involving patients should have ethics committee approval. Procedures for checking that this has been given before a trial begins should involve the administrator of the local research ethics committee, i.e. be independent of the local investigator or of a pharmacist committee member.

The regulatory status of the product under investigation should be checked and, whether or not there is a product licence, written confirmation should be seen that the necessary exemption and/or certificate has been received [20]. Substances without a product licence require an exemption certificate and, for medicines with a product licence, an exemption letter is issued (Table 3.1). For a doctor or dentist wishing to carry out his/her own clinical trial on a licensed product but where, for example, the dose, route or indication is

Table 3.1   Clinical trial exemption documents

CTC	CTX	DDX
Clinical trial certificate	Clinical trial exemption certificate	Doctor or dentist exemption certificate
Permits the use of a medicine in a trial	Permits the use of a medicine in a trial without having a CTC. Most trials undertaken using this	Permits a practitioner to undertake a non-commercial trial

not covered by the product licence, a doctor or dentist exemption certificate (DDX) is required.

Pharmacy should have a copy of all trial protocols, including codes, for studies in either the hospital or community services [2]. Arrangements need to be made for breaking any codes in an emergency. A useful checklist for other information which may be required on setting up a trial has been published, but regulatory status must be added to it [21]. Advice on the patient's eligibility for prescription charges is given in Department of Health letter DS21/75, quoted in the Royal Pharmaceutical Society of Great Britain guidelines, currently being updated.

All medicines, or constituent ingredients, for clinical trials should be ordered, stored and dispensed by the hospital pharmacy. Separate stocks should not be kept elsewhere in the hospital. Accurate records must be maintained of receipt, dispensing, issue, administration and disposal and 'regularly audited by pharmacy staff, with reconciliation, where necessary' [2]. Disposal of unused products in a company-sponsored trial must be according to the company's instructions. A computer system, CLINTIS, has been developed to help with pharmacy administration of trials [22].

Charges for work done in support of clinical trials are a difficult issue but are required if the pharmacy is to give the necessary support without detriment to the normal service [23]. For example, an on-call clinical trials team of pharmacy technicians was established with an estimated 30% of the funding from fees charged to pharmaceutical companies [24].

The future

Inpatient medicine supply systems have involved considerable time, space and stock-holding in the pharmacy to reduce the quantity supplied to the ward from that available in the manufacturer's bulk or outer pack. The trend towards use of manufacturers' original packs allows a fundamental rethink of how the pharmacy operates.

A number of hospitals, most notably Perth, have developed a ward order assembly agreement with a wholesaler [25]. Hospital pharmacy staff use hand-held terminals to scan ward stocks. These data are compared with the stock list and requirements calculated automatically, then sent via electronic data interchange to the wholesaler. Orders are despatched labelled for the ultimate destination, eliminating rehandling costs in hospital. Savings in space, stock and time have been reported but it is not yet certain what the charges will be if such a service is widely adopted and there is an inherent risk in one supplier having a virtual monopoly. Making use of the wholesaler's investment in automation and, for peripheral hospitals without a pharmacy, its transport, is logical, though moves to one-stop dispensing are reducing ward stock requirements.

Pneumatic conveying (air tube) systems are being increasingly used for rapid delivery of ward stock and discharge medicines within a hospital. Until electronic prescribing is more widely available (see chapter 11), time and effort are saved by sending prescriptions to pharmacy this way. They can help to support pharmacy staff who are working in a decentralised, clinically based system [26]. The only problem may be if the system fails, if delivery is not then necessarily to the intended destination.

Automation is becoming more feasible with the availability of robotic systems handling patient packs, now an integral part of modern practice [27]. A product requested through the pharmacy computer system for issue as ward stock or for dispensing can be automatically selected using the pack's bar code. The pack is delivered, within 15 seconds of the request being made, via a conveyor belt to the appropriate chute in the dispensing area, which can be sited adjacent to the terminal where the dispensing label is printed to minimise opportunity for error. Wastage is minimised as items with the shortest expiry dates are selected first. Scanning of bar codes is also used in loading such machines, enabling the robot to identify different products, strengths or pack sizes. When a pack is placed on the entry conveyor the dimensions are measured electronically so that the robot's computer can allocate an appropriate space. Products can be packed very compactly because any gaps can be filled without regard to any human need for selection, positions being memorised by the system's computer. The whole machine can also occupy less floor space than an equivalent amount of conventional shelving as the full floor to ceiling height (up to 3 metres) can be utilised.

The Audit Commission report cites one of the benefits of installing a robotic system at Wirral Hospital as being a reduction of reported dispensing errors from 19 to 7 per 100 000 items [16]. The previous error rate is comparable to the 16.3 and 17.6 per 100 000 items reported from other hospitals [28]. Other benefits included reduced dispensary turnaround times, simplified ordering systems, improved reliability of service and more efficient use of staff. It is therefore evident that, at least for the dispensing function, such automated systems fulfil all the criteria required of the medicine supply process.

References

1. NHS Executive Controls Assurance Standard on Medicines Management, Revision 02 (2001). http://www.open.gov.uk/doh/riskman.htm (accessed 12 May 2002).
2. Department of Health. *Guidelines for the Safe and Secure Handling of Medicines: A Report to the Secretary of State for Social Services – The Duthie Report*. London: Department of Health, 1988.
3. Department of Health and Social Security. *Report on Control of Dangerous Drugs and Poisons in Hospital – The Aitken Report*. London: HMSO, 1958.
4. Baker J A. Recent developments in the pharmaceutical service at Westminster Hospital. *J Hosp Pharm* 1967; 24: 400–406.
5. Calder G, Barnett J W. The pharmacist in the ward. *Pharm J* 1967; 198: 584–586.
6. The Hospital Pharmacists Group. One-stop dispensing, use of patients' own drugs and self-administration schemes. *Hosp Pharm* 2002; 9: 81–86.
7. Jeffery L. 28 day patient pack discharge medication. *Pharm Manage* 2001; 17: 24–25.
8. Semple J S, Morgan J E, Garner S T *et al*. The effect of self-administration and reuse of patients' own drugs on a hospital pharmacy. *Pharm J* 1995; 255: 124–126.
9. Cousins D H, Upton D R. Take care when using PODs. *Pharm Pract* 1998; 8: 26–32.
10. Ellis S, Ford P M, Hetherington C *et al*. Unit dose drug distribution at the Hospital for Women, Leeds. *Pharm J* 1973; 211: 276–278.
11. NHS Executive. *Responsibility for Prescribing Between GPs and Hospitals*. EL(91)127. London: NHS Executive, 1991.
12. Barker A. 28-day outpatient dispensing – only a simple step? *Pharm Manage* 2002; 18: 11–13.
13. Ashton C. How can we improve outpatient waiting times? *Hosp Pharm* 1999; 6: 115–118.
14. Department of Health. *The Way Forward for Hospital Pharmaceutical Services*. HC(88)54. London: Department of Health, 1988.

15. National Assembly for Wales. *Report of the Task and Finish Group on Prescribing*, 2000.
16. Audit Commission. *A Spoonful of Sugar – Medicines Management in NHS Hospitals*. London: Audit Commission, 2001.
17. *Misuse of Drugs Regulations 2001*. London: The Stationery Office, 2001.
18. *Misuse of Drugs Regulations (Safe Custody) 1973*. SI no. 798. London: The Stationery Office, 1973.
19. Cousins D H, Upton D R. Is it time to make strong KCl a controlled drug? *Pharm Pract* 2000; 10: 187.
20. Wiffen P J. A guide to the licensing system. *Hosp Pharm* 1995; 2: 15–16.
21. Jacklin A, Schwartz B, Barber N. Checklist for clinical trials. *Br J Pharm Pract* 1988; 10: 352.
22. McDonald A, Hume A. Managing clinical trials – organising chaos? *Pharm Manage* 1998; 14: 15–17.
23. Hewetson M L, Root T. Charging for clinical trials. *Hosp Pharm* 1995; 2: 19–21.
24. News item. Guy's sets up on-call clinical team. *Hosp Pharm* 1997; 4: 165.
25. Low J, Radley A, Dodd T *et al.* Ward order assembly – 'just in time'. *Hosp Pharm* 1998; 5: 109–112.
26. Bunn R J, Tyrell A M, Thomas M K. Restructuring hospital pharmacy services on 'patient focussed care' principles – three years on. *Hosp Pharm* 1997; 4: 158–162.
27. Gross Z. Robotic dispensing device installed at St Thomas's Hospital. *Pharm J* 2000; 265: 653–655.
28. Spencer M G, Smith A P. A multicentre study of dispensing errors in NHS hospitals. *Pharm. J* 1992; 249: (suppl. R14).

Further reading

Barnett J W. Supply of medicines. In: Allwood M C, Fell J T, ed. *Textbook of Hospital Pharmacy*. Oxford: Blackwell, 1980: 277–330.

Department of Health. *Guidelines for the Safe and Secure Handling of Medicines: A Report to the Secretary of State for Social Services – 'The Duthie Report'*. London: Department of Health, 1988.

The Hospital Pharmacists Group. One-stop dispensing, use of patients' own drugs and self-administration schemes. *Hosp Pharm* 2002; 9: 81–86.

4

Technical services

Graham Sewell

The term 'technical services' usually refers to the elements of hospital pharmacy organisational structure related to pharmaceutical production and manufacturing. The definition has been modified to suit local situations and changes in emphasis within hospital pharmacy production and preparation. For the purposes of this chapter, technical services will include:

- pharmaceutical repackaging
- non-sterile manufacturing
- sterile manufacturing (terminal sterilisation)
- aseptic preparation, including:
  — parenteral infusions
  — cytotoxic infusions
  — total parenteral nutrition (TPN) solutions
  — radiopharmaceuticals.

In some centres, the different aspects of aseptic preparation are grouped under the heading Centralised Intravenous Additive Services (CIVAS). However, this does not adequately describe aseptic preparations requiring more complex manipulations than simple addition or the preparation of parenteral products for non-intravenous administration.

This chapter will outline the historical development of technical services and then describe current practice in the different aspects listed above. The responsiveness of technical services to clinical need and changes in practice are illustrated with selected examples of development and progress. These also serve to emphasise the interdependence of hospital pharmacy clinical and technical services. Finally, the new challenges facing technical services will be explored in the context of future trends in health care services.

History

In the last 30 years, the focus of production and repackaging activities in hospital pharmacies has changed dramatically. In the early 1970s, it was common practice for even small district general hospitals (DGHs) to engage in a wide range of production activities. Non-sterile production would have typically included a range of oral liquids and mixtures (often preserved with chloroform water), antiseptic skin-staining solutions for use in theatre, suppositories, creams, ointments and powders. Many of the formulae for these products were obtained from the official literature such as the *British Pharmaceutical Codex*, although a number of formulations were 'developed' in-house [1]. Topical preparations for dermatology clinics were often particularly challenging, with many containing coal tar preparations. In the absence of a commercially available product at the time, dilutions of topical steroids (e.g. Betnovate cream, 1 in 4 dilution) were also prepared.

Many hospitals had also realised the benefits of preparing stocks of commonly used solid-dosage forms as prepacks on a small-batch scale. These become known as 'ward packs' and were prepared using manual (e.g. tablet triangle) or semiautomatic tablet/capsule-counting systems. Labels were often preprinted and batch-specific details were either hand-written or typed.

With few exceptions, non-sterile manufacturing and prepacking occurred on an ad hoc, small-scale basis, with little central coordination. Batch records, procedures and production facilities were all extremely variable and little thought was given to process validation, shelf-life assignment, quality assurance (QA) and control.

The manufacture of terminally sterilised products was also more widespread in the 1970s than is currently the case. The presence of small autoclaves, dry-heat sterilisers and steam baths was common in DGH pharmacies, and many hospitals were self-sufficient in their provision of most sterile products, buying only the 'bulk' intravenous (IV) infusions (e.g. 0.9% sodium chloride and 5% glucose) from industry. The product range typically included bladder irrigation solutions, multidose eye drops, antiseptic solutions and oily preparations for sterile wound dressings. In some centres, specialist injectables for IV, intramuscular (IM) and intrathecal administration were also produced.

In most cases, bulk solutions were prepared in uncontrolled or perhaps socially clean areas and were invariably filled into glass containers which were sealed with a rubber stopper and screw-cap arrangement. A basic filtration procedure was usually incorporated for parenteral products and eye drops and some of the more specialised units had ampoule sealing equipment, which was normally semiautomatic at best. Sterilisation processes were poorly controlled and rarely validated, particularly in the case of steam baths (for heating with a bactericide) and dry-heat sterilisers. Quality control (QC) was usually rudimentary, with only an inspection of the product for visible particulates and an examination of sterilisation cycle temperature–time charts prior to batch release.

As the decade of the 1970s progressed, sterile production did become more organised with the emergence of specialist sterile product units on a coordinated, regional basis. Many of these units concentrated on the production of sterile large-volume irrigation solutions which were normally presented in semirigid plastic containers (e.g. Schubert containers). These units benefited from considerable investment to fund automatic filling lines, hermetic sealing technology and large double-ended autoclaves. A few UK centres were equipped to fill flexible-film polyvinyl chloride (PVC) containers for the manufacture of large-volume IV infusions and small blow-moulded containers for eye drops.

By comparison with sterile and non-sterile manufacturing, aseptic preparation was a relatively minor component of hospital pharmacy work in the mid-1970s. The Breckenridge Report was published in 1976 and recognised the hazards of infusion preparation on hospital wards [2]. This prompted the development of embryonic CIVAS in a few of the larger teaching hospitals, which prepared TPN and other solutions which were considered of insufficient stability to withstand terminal sterilisation processes. As with other types of hospital production of the era, facilities, controls and documentation were often neglected. The preparation of radiopharmaceuticals at the time was largely confined to nuclear medicine departments, where the work was carried out by medical physics staff under the supervision of medical staff.

An attempt to rationalise hospital technical services activities through the introduction of rigorous costing policies was made in 1984 with the issue of health circular HC(84)3 by the Department of Health [3]. This circular recommended that hospitals should not produce pharmaceuticals which were commercially available and that the economic viability of in-house manufacture should be assessed. This included taking into account the full cost of facilities, equipment, maintenance, heating, lighting and depreciation when calculating the cost of products. At the time, this health circular was not well received by technical services pharmacists and, apart from encouraging further rationalisation through regional production units, its impact was limited.

Of much greater significance was the loss from National Health Service (NHS) hospitals of Crown immunity in 1990. Under new guidelines manufacturing activities above specified levels were required to be licensed by the Medicines Control Agency (MCA) [4]. For many smaller production units, the cost of upgrading facilities to the standards required to obtain a MCA 'specials' manufacturing licence was prohibitive. The loss of Crown immunity coincided with the introduction of trust status for many NHS hospitals. The combination of new, higher standards and a more cost-conscious environment in the NHS significantly changed the emphasis of technical services activities. More recently, the issue of Guidance Note 14 [5] and enthusiastic enforcement by the MCA have effectively eliminated products made under a manufacturing specials licence where a licensed equivalent is available. This has led to concerns about intellectual property rights of hospital-developed formulations which can be copied by industry and sold back to the NHS at high cost in a protected market. This new guidance also prevents hospital manufacturing units responding to supply problems, which seem increasingly prevalent in the pharmaceutical industry.

Licensing issues

With the exception of a limited number of lines produced by specialist hospital manufacturing units, medicines produced by hospital technical services departments are unlicensed and have no product licence (PL) or marketing authorisation. If the production of an unlicensed medicine is conducted under the supervision of a pharmacist, and the batch size and frequency of preparation are within MCA-defined limits, Section 10 of the 1968 Medicines Act provides exemption from the requirement to hold a manufacturer's licence [4]. Apart from the above limitations, manufacture under Section 10 exemption prohibits supply of the product outside the NHS trust in which it was made and imposes limits on the maximum shelf-life which may be assigned to certain product types.

For the production of larger batches and in the case of medicines sold outside the production unit's trust, a manufacturer's specials licence is required. The specials licence is regulated by the MCA and permits the manufacture of products which are not subject to a PL. The licence specifies the type of manufacture permitted (e.g. non-sterile, aseptic manufacture, etc.) and the product categories to which the licence applies (large-volume IVs, antibiotics, cytotoxics, biologicals, etc.). Hospitals holding a specials licence are subjected to regular audits by the MCA, including an inspection of facilities and a full audit of good manufacturing practice (GMP), QA and QC systems. Advertising of products manufactured under a specials licence is not permitted, although it is permissible to advertise a specials manufacturing service.

Repackaging (prepacking, assembly)

Scope

Repackaging is a process in which liquid or solid-dose formulations are packed from bulk into smaller, ready-to-use containers (prepacks). The presentation of prepacks, in terms of the number of tablets/capsules or volume of liquid, the label details and the container type, are designed to meet a specific clinical need. Until the mid-1990s, the most common repackaging activity undertaken by hospital pharmacy departments was the production of ward packs. Bulk packs of tablets and capsules (e.g. 500–5000 dose units) and large containers of liquid medicines (up to 2 litres) were economic to purchase, particularly from manufacturers of generics. However, it was neither economical nor pharmaceutically acceptable to place such large containers on hospital wards as stock medicines. Therefore ward packs were produced by repacking bulk medicines into pack sizes of typically 25–50 solid-dose units per pack or 50–200 ml of liquid medicines per bottle.

Repackaging also provided an opportunity to improve the clarity of labelling. The proprietary or trade name of the medicine was often prominent on bulk packs but the prepacks could be labelled with the approved name of the medicine to reduce the risk of drug administration errors on the ward.

In recent years the increased availability of commercially produced ward packs which carry a full UK PL (marketing authorisation) has reduced the need for in-house production of ward packs. Also the introduction of patient packs containing strips of blister-packed tablets and capsules has provided another presentation which can be adapted for ward use by simply overlabelling the outer carton. Although there will be a continued demand for a limited range of ward packs which are not commercially available, the emphasis of hospital repackaging activities is directed towards more patient-specific packs which are not commercially viable. These include prepacks for hospital discharge medication and packs designed to meet the requirements of specific treatment protocols or patient group directives in primary, secondary and tertiary care settings. The objective in both cases is to produce a presentation which exactly meets specific clinical and patient requirements while minimising repetitive, labour-intensive dispensing work. The MCA provides guidance on the requirement for a special assembly licence for repackaging, depending on the batch size and the frequency with which batches are produced [4]. Increasingly, hospital repackaging is becoming centralised in specialist units with automated packing lines. Although repackaging whole strips of blister-packed medicines into different containers is acceptable, the removal of tablets or capsules from blisters for repackaging is not advisable since stability cannot be guaranteed.

Facilities and equipment

In its simplest form, repackaging is a manual operation in which counting of tablets/capsules and measuring of liquids are achieved with tablet triangles, capsule trays and glass measures. Containers are also capped and labelled by hand, although all labels are either preprinted or produced on a computer labelling system. Repackaging activities require a clean, uncluttered, designated area. Walls, floors and work surfaces should be of a smooth, impervious finish and should be readily accessible for easy cleaning. Although most tablets are now coated, dust containing active drug can be generated during repackaging and a localised dust extraction system should be fitted.

The degree of automation of repackaging processes ranges from semiautomatic tablet and capsule-counting machines to fully automated packing lines. In the case of the latter, empty containers are sorted, oriented and then transported to the filling zone by a conveyor track. Tablets or capsules are fed from a hopper over a chip-sieve to counting heads, which fill the correct number of dose units into each container. The containers progress to an automated capping system before preprinted labels are applied automatically. Many packing lines are fitted with localised dust extraction in critical areas and also electronic check-weight systems to assure correct counting and filling processes. An example of a fully automatic packing line is shown in Figure 4.1. This type of equipment must be easily dismantled and reassembled to permit cleaning and inspection between batch runs.

Process

Repackaging processes are simple but errors can occur. To avoid transposition of medicines or labels it is essential that only one batch is

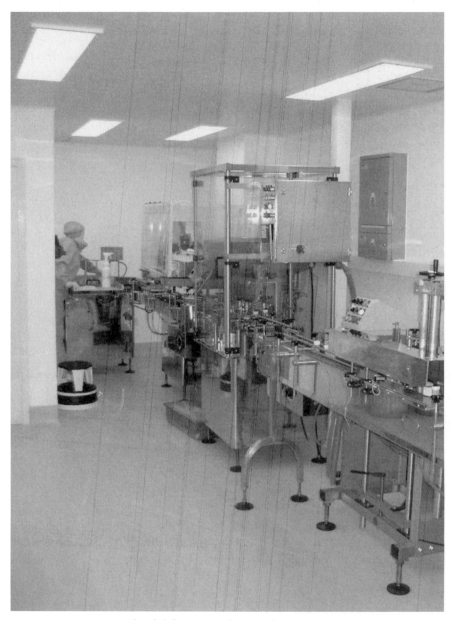

Figure 4.1 Automated solid-dose repackaging line at Royal Devon and Exeter Hospital.

repackaged at a time in a designated area and that the work area is cleared of all labels, containers and medicines from the previous batch. With solid-dose forms, it is good practice to organise the repackaging schedule so that medicines differ from the previous batch repackaged in colour, shape, size or appearance. This makes it easier to detect the odd 'rogue' tablet or capsule transposed to another batch of a different product in error.

It is also important that cleaning procedures for equipment are carefully validated, particularly if sensitising antibiotics such as penicillins are repackaged, to ensure that medicines are not contaminated with dust from previous batches.

When repackaging liquids (particularly suspensions) it is essential to shake the bulk container thoroughly before distributing the liquid to the prepack containers. This ensures that the concentration of drug in all prepacked containers is homogeneous. In practice, these processes are controlled through standard operating procedures, batch documentation, staff training and competency assessment. The reconciliation of the number of dose units used, the number of packs produced and the number of labels issued and used all require particular consideration. These controls should be part of a comprehensive QA system, which will also include QC, self-inspection, error reporting and feedback from 'customers'.

Non-sterile manufacture

Scope

The manufacture of traditional non-sterile oral liquids and topical preparations, usually in accordance with *British Pharmaceutical Codex* formulae [1], has declined in the hospital sector over recent years. This is largely due to the commercial availability of licensed products and also the growth of non-sterile specials manufacturing services.

However, a non-sterile production service is still required to support several clinical specialities, particularly dermatology and paediatrics. Many dermatologists have their own variants of standard preparations, often differing only in the type of diluent or base used or in the concentration of active components. Although there is little scientific evidence to support the use of these non-standard preparations, custom, practice and clinical experience provide a continuing demand.

Conversely, the clinical justification for using medicines outside their licensed indications for adults in the paediatric setting is well

accepted. The unit dose of commercially available preparations of medicines designed for adult use is usually too large for paediatrics. Also,
some of the larger tablets and capsules would be difficult for children to
swallow. Safe and reproducible paediatric dosing therefore requires
preparations of lower dose, usually oral liquids, suspensions or
powders.

A recent Department of Health report suggests that dermatology
preparations (coal tar, salicylic acid and dithranol) remain the most frequently prepared non-sterile products by hospital pharmacy departments [6]. Some hospitals have developed commercial non-sterile
manufacturing units to supply other hospitals and community pharmacies. This type of activity helps to offset the costs of maintaining facilities of a high standard and meeting the regulatory requirements of
manufacturers' specials licences.

In some hospitals, dispensary services have been reorganised and
extemporaneous dispensing work has been transferred to the technical
services section. A wide range of non-commercially available extemporaneous preparations is required for individual patients, including oral
liquids, creams, ointments, powders, suppositories and pessaries. This
approach provides variety and clinical interest for manufacturing staff
and ensures that extemporaneous products are produced in accordance
with the principles of GMP.

Facilities and equipment

Typically, non-sterile manufacture is carried out in a European Union
(EU) grade-D environment with a single stage change [7]. Although
some units require production staff to wear sterilised coverall gowns,
most centres rely on clean, two-piece gowns of low-lint-shedding material, overshoes, hats and gloves. To reduce the microbiological bioburden, drains and potable water supplies are excluded from production
areas and all surfaces should have a smooth impervious finish to facilitate effective cleaning. Weighing areas should be separate from the main
production area (linked to it with a pass-through hatch) and should be
fitted with localised dust extraction. Although containers for non-sterile
products are not reused, a facility for washing and drying containers
before use may be required. Separate areas should be provided for
labelling and reinspection of products.

The *Rules and Guidance for Good Pharmaceutical Manufacture
and Distribution* strongly recommends the use of stainless-steel measures and mixing vessels to avoid the risk of contaminating product with

spicules from glass equipment [7]. Large-scale manufacture will require the use of industrial mixers and homogenisers. Automated liquid filling lines may be deployed for large-scale liquid handling and some units with a significant output of creams and ointments have also invested in tube-filling and sealing equipment. Figure 4.2 illustrates small-scale non-sterile manufacturing facilities.

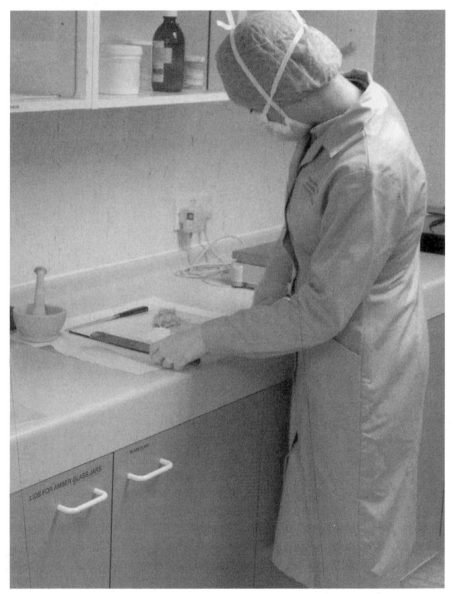

Figure 4.2 Small-scale non-sterile manufacturing at Derriford Hospital, Plymouth.

Process

All raw materials, containers and labels used in the production process must be approved by the person responsible for QC. To reduce the microbiological bioburden, limits are placed on the level of microbiological contamination of raw materials and only sterile water (usually water for irrigation BP) or freshly distilled water is used for manufacture. All product formulae, storage conditions and shelf-life assignments require prior QC approval.

The manufacturing process is controlled through the use of approved standard operating procedures and batch documents of work sheets. Particular care is required to ensure that mixing processes produce a homogeneous product for distribution into the individual containers that constitute the batch. This process must be validated for each product type to ensure uniformity of content in the finished batch.

The avoidance of cross-contamination between different products is also essential. Only one batch may be prepared in a designated work area at any one time and the cleaning of equipment and work surfaces must be carefully validated and monitored.

Filled containers should be visually inspected for product homogeneity and the absence of any extraneous matter. The security of container closures should be checked and the quality and accuracy of labels determined against a master label for the product. It is essential that the batch documentation includes a reconciliation between the amounts of raw materials, number of containers and number of labels used in the process and the yield of finished product. All variations must be recorded and investigated.

Sterile manufacture

Scope

All terminally sterilised medicines produced in hospitals are made under a manufacturer's specials licence, except in a few cases where PLs have been obtained. The range of products made generally reflects gaps in the portfolio of licensed products available from the pharmaceutical industry. The limited number of specialist sterile manufacturing units remaining in the NHS provides an essential service in making available sterile parenteral and topical products that are not commercially viable for industry. Such products include non-standard concentrations and presentations of injections and eye drops, specialist injectables for paediatrics, anaesthetics and palliative care and various sterile topical products.

In some cases, NHS hospital sterile product units have developed products to support pharmacy CIVAS. These include electrolytes for addition to TPN feeds such as concentrated sodium chloride injection, potassium phosphate injection and zinc sulphate injection. A range of sterile bulk solutions for filling into syringes and other devices is also produced. These include bupivacaine injection, morphine sulphate injection and fentanyl injection. Sterile manufacture also supports research and small runs of experimental drugs in parenteral formulations are prepared for clinical trial use.

The container and filling technologies employed in hospital units encompass glass vials, glass ampoules, glass bottles and PVC infusion bags for parenteral products and a variety of glass and rigid plastic containers for topical solutions. No lyophilised presentations are available since freeze-drying technology is beyond the scope of hospital sterile product units.

Facilities and equipment

In general, the weighing and solution preparation areas required will be similar to those described previously for non-sterile manufacture. However, the filling, sealing and capping stages must be accomplished in a higher-quality environment, usually EU grade A, to minimise particulate contamination and reduce the microbiological load prior to sterilisation. This is usually achieved by local laminar air flow at the filling zone.

After filling and sealing, containers and their contents are sterilised by steam in an autoclave (aqueous solutions) or by dry heat in a hot-air oven (non-aqueous liquids, powders). The sterilisers and associated monitoring equipment can be located in a lower-grade environment and should be sited so that maintenance staff can access them without the need to enter critical production areas.

Dedicated space for reinspection of the finished product, labelling, packing and quarantine is also required. Regulatory requirements for sterile production facilities and sterilising equipment are strictly defined [7]. The design and construction of sterile manufacturing units should only be undertaken by specialist contractors.

The increasing use of automated systems, particularly for filling, sealing and reinspecting ampoules, and the sophistication of modern steriliser technology have contributed to the rapid rise in capital and maintenance costs associated with sterile manufacturing units. National coordination and strategic planning of new units are essential to maximise the cost-effectiveness of these expensive but important resources.

Process

In addition to the processes outlined under non-sterile manufacturing, sterile production normally includes a filtration process (for liquids) and sterilisation of the product. These processes are critical to product quality and require rigorous validation and control. The microbiological bioburden must be minimised, particularly in the case of injectables, to reduce the release of bacterial pyrogens into the product, which will not be destroyed by sterilisation. This is achieved by limiting the number of viable microorganisms in starting materials and by minimising the time between preparation of the bulk product, filling and sterilisation.

The sterilisation cycle for each batch is clearly monitored to ensure that all containers in the batch have received the pharmacopoeial-approved temperature and time combinations [8]. Printouts of the load temperature, usually taken at the coolest location of the autoclave or dry-heat oven, are recorded throughout the cycle and are scrutinised as part of the release process. Additional measures are taken to ensure that products sterilised by autoclave or hot-air oven are not at risk from microbial contamination of cooling water or non-sterile air, respectively, which could enter through closures during the cooling phase of

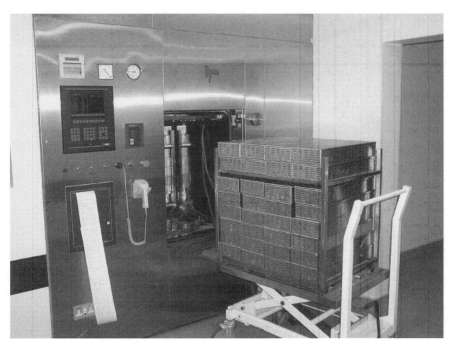

Figure 4.3   Autoclave at PMU, Torbay Hospital.

the cycle. Figure 4.3 shows an autoclave and its control systems in a large sterile production unit.

The QC of sterile products includes sterility testing, subvisual particulate measurement and tests for the absence of bacterial pyrogens. This means that batches must be quarantined for at least 14 days (the time taken for sterility test incubation) before release. Production managers and users of sterile products need to consider this when drawing up production schedules and managing stocks.

Aseptic preparation

Scope

Most aseptic preparation work undertaken in the hospital setting is described by the following categories:

- intravenous additions
- TPN
- cytotoxic infusions
- radiopharmaceuticals.

Stability issues frequently preclude the provision of 'ready-to-use' parenteral medicines by the pharmaceutical industry. Many drugs, including antibiotics, opioid analgesics and cytotoxics, are degraded by hydrolysis. In order to assign a reasonable shelf-life to these medicines, parenteral formulations are presented as lyophilised powders which require reconstitution (in some cases dilution) before administration to the patient. Aseptic manipulation is also necessary either for clinical reasons, in which doses or formulations need to be tailored for individual patients, or because stability issues preclude the provision of a 'ready-to-use' product by the pharmaceutical industry.

The same principles of aseptic preparation apply to all four categories, although there are subtle differences in the processes and equipment used for each product type. Many hospitals group the first three activities under the heading CIVAS, although others consider TPN and cytotoxic work to be separate.

Aseptic preparation work is a high-risk activity; the risk of calculation or compounding errors and the risk of microbiological contamination must be controlled to ensure the safety and efficacy of aseptic preparations. The UK CIVAS group conducted a national study on failure rates in media-fill simulations of aseptic processes and found this to be approximately 1 in 500 [9]. However these risks need to be placed in the context of the alternative to hospital pharmacy-based aseptic services. Although evidence is limited, intuitively it is clear that the risk of errors and microbiological contamination will be considerably higher if aseptic manipulations are carried out by untrained staff in clinical areas. Certainly the Audit Commission supported the use of CIVAS in its *A Spoonful of Sugar:* 'making up aseptic preparations in hospital wards should be stopped' [10].

Since the unfortunate deaths of children from contaminated parenteral nutrition solutions, the regulation of aseptic preparation has been strictly enforced by the UK Department of Health.

Hospitals preparing aseptic products under a specials manufacturing licence are subject to rigorous inspection and increasing demands by the Medicines Control Agency. Unlicensed units (those claiming Medicines Act section 10 exemption) must follow the guidance set out in *Aseptic Dispensing for NHS Patients* [11]. The authority for enforcing compliance with this document has been delegated to regional quality assurance pharmacists by the Department of Health. This document also restricts the shelf-life assigned to products produced in unlicensed facilities to a maximum of 7 days, irrespective of whether stability data would support a longer shelf-life.

Intravenous additives

Many medicines for parenteral administration are provided as concentrates or lyophilised powders. These require reconstitution and/or dilution followed by transfer to a device (such as a syringe) for administration to the patient. The need for pharmacy-based IV additive services was recognised in the Breckenridge report of 1976 [2]. However, recent studies in the north-west of England have shown that only 35% of medicines requiring aseptic manipulation are prepared by the hospital pharmacy department [12]. Most departments target high-risk areas for their services. These include the provision of paediatric doses of steroids, analgesics and antibiotics and also anaesthetic/analgesic combinations for epidural infusion. Many hospitals also provide subcutaneous infusions of drug combinations used in palliative care, as well as prefilled syringes to support patient-controlled analgesia. They also provide antibiotic infusions in disposable infusion devices for domiciliary patients with cystic fibrosis or osteomyelitis. A recent Department of Health survey placed infusions of morphine, bupivacaine, desferrioxamine and three antibiotics into the top 10 aseptic products produced by hospitals [6].

Total parenteral nutrition

Fewer hospitals are now preparing TPN solutions from scratch. Standardisation of regimens for adults, paediatrics and neonates has enabled commercial manufacturers with specials licences to take a significant part of the TPN market. Also new technologies such as multi-compartmental TPN bags enable manufacturers to provide macronutrients in standard quantities as terminally sterilised solutions in individual compartments of the bag. These presentations have long shelf-lives, often at room temperature, and are activated to permit mixing of components immediately before use. Many of the hospitals where TPN is still compounded prepare batches of 'base-TPN' bags in which macronutrients (glucose, amino acids, lipid and water) are present in standard amounts. Standard TPN formulations are available with standard electrolyte concentrations or as electrolyte-free solutions to which patient-specific electrolytes can be added before administration. In all cases, it is necessary to add unstable components such as vitamins and trace elements prior to use.

Standard formulae are satisfactory for the majority of patients requiring TPN and there is no scientific or clinical evidence to support some of the very complex individualised preparations that have been used. It must be recognised, however, that some patients (e.g. renal patients) have specific needs and the NHS must retain the expertise and capacity to compound individualised TPN feeds in cases of genuine clinical need.

Cytotoxics

The risk of occupational exposure to these mutagenic and potentially carcinogenic drugs has restricted the preparation of all cytotoxic doses to specialist facilities in the hospital pharmacy. The narrow therapeutic index, extreme toxicity and complex regimens of cytotoxics provide strong clinical reasons for dose calculation and preparation by experienced staff using well-controlled systems. A close working relationship between clinical pharmacy and technical services staff is desirable for all aseptic work, but is essential in the case of cytotoxics.

Pressures on pharmacy cytotoxic services include increased demand as more cancer patients receive chemotherapy and also an increasing trend towards outpatient-based administration of chemotherapy. This places immediate demands on the service to avoid lengthy patient waiting times and the risk of errors caused by untrained staff administering chemotherapy outside normal working hours. Strategies designed to offset these pressures include dose-banding, which enables doses to be prepared as standard prefilled syringes which are used in combination to provide the 'banded' dose [13]. This approach is, of course, dependent upon the stability of the reconstituted infusions. The advent of gene therapy and targeted therapy using antibiotics and viral vectors will add to the challenge faced by oncology pharmacy services.

Radiopharmaceuticals

Nuclear medicine provides important diagnostic and functional information on specific organs in addition to radiation therapy for certain disease states. Diagnostic scans are used in many specialities including oncology, cardiology, surgery, neurology and renal medicine. Departments routinely perform investigations such as cardiac scans to evaluate the extent of heart disease, bone scans to detect metastatic disease and cell labelling to help evaluate whether infectious or non-infectious inflammatory conditions are present. As radiation detectors continue to improve and new ligands are developed, the number of clinical applications continues to expand. Lymph scanning is a case in point where technological advances have now enabled surgeons to use the scan to assist in staging of malignant melanomas and breast cancer.

Radiopharmacy is a specialised area of CIVAS with several unique characteristics. Radiopharmaceuticals have extremely short shelf-lives compared to other pharmaceuticals. Shelf-lives are frequently measured in the range of seconds, hours and days rather than weeks, months or years, and this requires that doses are prepared on the day of use using radionuclides obtained freshly from a technetium generator kept in the radiopharmacy.

Facilities and equipment

All aseptic manipulation must take place in EU grade-A work zones [7]. These can be provided by horizontal or vertical laminar air flow cabinets or positive-pressure isolators. For hazardous drugs, such as cytotoxics and radiopharmaceuticals, the use of a negative-pressure isolator is recommended to provide protection not only to the product, but also the operator(s) [14]. The grade-A workstation must be located in a controlled background environment, usually of EU grade B, although some isolators may be located in an EU grade-C or D background. Figure 4.4 shows horizontal laminar flow workstations used for IV additive work.

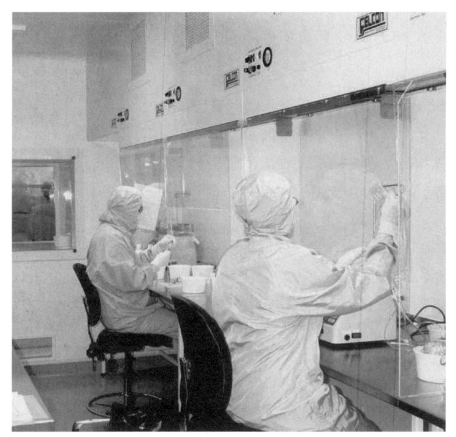

Figure 4.4 Aseptic compounding in laminar air flow workstation at ASU, University of Bath.

Automated filling equipment may be placed in the critical work zone. Figure 4.5 shows an Automix system for compounding TPN solutions.

The *Rules and Guidance for Good Pharmaceutical Manufacture and Distribution* [7] and *Quality Assurance of Aseptic Preparation Services* [15] should be consulted for exact standards and requirements of facilities and equipment. Specialist guidance on isolator technology is also available [16].

In addition to the critical aseptic handling areas, areas must be designated for setting up ingredients, producing batch documents and labels and checking and packing the finished product. Handling radio-pharmaceuticals requires additional equipment to protect the operator

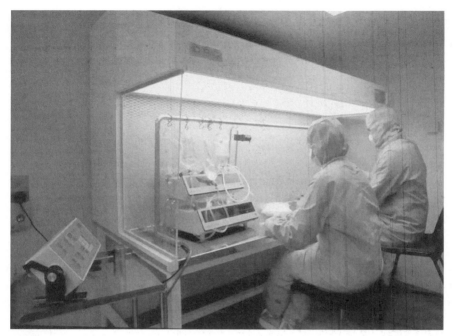

Figure 4.5 Total parenteral nutrition compounding using Baxter Automix system at Derriford Hospital, Plymouth.

from ionising radiation and to monitor exposure levels. Also, tandem isolator systems are necessary to include the technetium (Tc99) generator in the controlled work area (Figure 4.6). Operators are required to wear body badges and finger badges in order to quantify the amount of exposure they have received. They must also follow systems of work which control exposure by either minimising the time spent directly exposed to the source of radiation or by maximising the distance from it. Such practices include working behind lead glass shields and the use of syringe and vial shields and lead housing for generators. These shields must also be accommodated within the isolator or class 2 cabinet workstation. Tongs are used to increase the distance between the operator and the doses. Dose monitors are also used to check for spillages and contamination and are subsequently used to ensure such incidents are cleared up appropriately. There are specific elements of operator training which must be covered besides the routine pharmacy training. There are also 'local rules' which must be read which cover the safe systems of working with radiation.

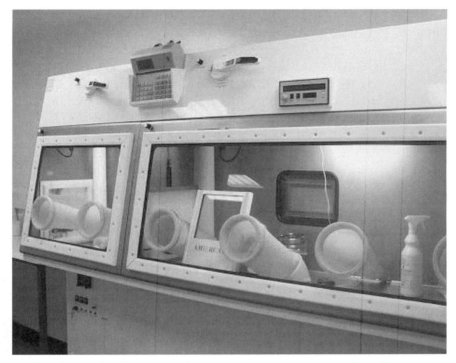

Figure 4.6 Radiopharmacy workstation at St George's Hospital, London.

Process

Wherever possible, all aseptic processes should be based on closed systems so that the product or the product fluid path has only minimal exposure to the environment. Product segregation is essential to prevent gross contamination and separate clean rooms and workstations should be used for cytotoxic drugs and radiopharmaceuticals. Operator technique is critical and all operators, processes and equipment must be fully validated.

The manipulation of cytotoxic drugs requires additional protective clothing and emergency procedures for spillage management. These are detailed in non-official UK guidelines [14, 17]. To avoid aerosol formation, venting needles and filters must be used when adding and withdrawing liquids to and from vials.

In the case of aseptic products, environmental monitoring and the use of routine media-fill simulations are more meaningful than sterility tests used with terminally sterilised medicines. Support from an experienced QA department is essential not only for the validation of all aseptic processes but also for formulation and shelf-life issues with aseptic preparations.

The additional risks associated with intrathecal administration of cytotoxic agents have led to additional guidance on process and release of these products – the aim being to prevent the lethal intrathecal administration of vinca alkaloids [18]. The processes involved in the preparation of radiopharmaceuticals require consideration of additional issues, including the prescribing and scheduling of doses, which are often complex. Most doctors who request scans are not authorised to prescribe radioactive pharmaceuticals. Requests must therefore be authorised by the local Administration of Radioactive Substances Advisory Committee (ARSAC) licence holder before they can be scheduled into the nuclear medicine clinic. To maximise the scanning capacity of a nuclear medicine department, doses need to be ready at the beginning of the working day. An on-site radiopharmacy can help facilitate this and enable the service to be more flexible when responding to urgent requests. In contrast to routine CIVAS work, radiopharmacy staff commence dose preparation first thing in the morning and early starts of 7 a.m. are not unusual. Reconstitution of kits requires the addition of a radionuclide and saline to a ligand contained in a sterile vial. The resulting solution may need to be incubated for a set period to ensure the radionuclide has attached to the ligand. Some kits are boiled to ensure the required radiopharmaceutical is obtained. Simple QC analysis can be performed to confirm the radiochemical purity of the radiopharmaceutical. Poor-quality radiopharmaceuticals may expose patients to radiation unnecessarily and their treatment may be delayed while the investigation is repeated.

Education and training for hospital technical services

Technical services departments are expected to develop in-house training schemes for all grades of staff which fully cover all activities undertaken. All training must be fully documented and evidence of effectiveness of training must be supported by competency assessment. Observation of individual practice as a part of self-inspection schemes and operator validation data are important components of the assessment process. Training programmes should be reviewed regularly and updated in line with service and individual needs. Systems should be in place to identify staff who fail validation tests or are associated with poor QA monitoring data and repeated errors. Such individuals may need additional training and reassessment.

A number of formal education and training courses specialising in the pharmaceutical technical services are available in the UK. These include various short courses in specialised areas and postgraduate programmes leading to diploma or masters qualification. The Technical Specialist Education and Training (TSET) website is an excellent source of information for all types of courses: www.tset.org.uk.

Health and safety and environmental issues

In recent years, health care professionals have become increasingly aware of health risks in the workplace, partly because of the introduction of the *Control of Substances Hazardous to Health Regulations* [19]. In the case of technical services, particular risks identified relate to occupational exposure of hazardous materials, including solvents and powders used in classical manufacturing processes and cytotoxics and sensitising antibiotics handled by aseptic units. New pharmaceutical developments such as targeted toxins, gene therapy and viral vectors for drug delivery are entering clinical use. These new agents will present a particular challenge in aseptic preparation where measures to reduce or eliminate the risk of occupational exposure and cross-contamination of products must be adopted and validated.

Environmental issues are of increasing significance. Controls to prevent the discharge into the environment of genetic material, biologicals and radioactive substances are likely to become more stringent at a time when the medicinal use of such agents continues to increase. Collaborative research to develop safe handling and containment systems is essential, together with other measures to reduce the amounts of medical and plastic waste produced by the technical services activities.

The future

This section briefly considers some of the challenges faced by technical services and is intended to stimulate debate and discussion on the future of the service within the new NHS.

Competing pressures of resource limitations, staffing issues, workload volume and complexity and regulatory controls require a clear, coherent strategy for the organisation and development of technical services.

Clinical manufacturing activities (non-sterile and sterile manufacture) appear particularly vulnerable despite ongoing supply difficulties experienced by the pharmaceutical industry. Under local trust management, the remaining classical manufacturing units seem either to struggle for investment and resource or, conversely, are viewed purely as income-generation activities from which year-on-year increases in profit are required. This approach can only lead to increased costs of specials medicines for the NHS as a whole, inadequate capacity and the selection of product lines according to profitability rather than clinical need. Bungled local management has already resulted in the closure of excellent manufacturing units and the loss of valuable expertise from the NHS. Perhaps it is time to take this vital service under national rather than local control to support strategic planning and foster the cooperation required to provide a product portfolio based on clinical need rather than short-term profit.

Aseptic services have faced significant workload increases and, despite some welcome innovations by the pharmaceutical industry, this trend is likely to continue. In terms of contribution to direct clinical care, pharmacy aseptic services rank alongside medical imaging, laboratory services, theatres and outpatient departments. The challenge faced by hospital pharmacy managers is to ensure that trusts recognise the value of aseptic services and resource them accordingly. Staff shortages have restricted the development of aseptic services in some areas. It is likely that recruitment of staff outside the traditional pharmacy disciplines is the only solution. This approach would need the provision of specific training programmes, ideally developed nationally with input from relevant stakeholders, but delivered at local or regional level. The use of computer-aided learning technology could, at least in part, assist with this.

The availability of a comprehensive range of medicinal products, in clinically required presentations at affordable cost, is dependent upon a constructive and open relationship between hospital technical services departments and the pharmaceutical and medical device industries. Some national special interest groups have already recognised this. For example, the UK National CIVAS Group has always encouraged industry to provide 'ready-to-use' products. This is partly to help control the workload faced by hospital aseptic services and also because the Group supports the use of licensed products if they are available. The issue of Guidance Note 14 by the Medicines Control Agency [5] has not helped relations with industry. This document unwittingly supports the exploitation of hospital-led developments by industry for commercial gain. To protect against this, technical services pharmacists must recognise the value of intellectual property rights (IPR) in their developmental work. Revenue raised from the sale of IPR to industry could support further developmental activity and infrastructure.

The introduction and use of new technology in technical services are, in most parts of the UK, fragmented and uncoordinated. As a result, many aspects of the work, particularly in aseptic preparation, remain labour-intensive because the computer and robotic technologies required are either non-existent or poorly developed. Greater cooperation between centres on specification, development and investment strategies will be required before the full benefits of the new technologies can be realised.

Acknowledgement

The author is grateful to Maria Connelly (ASU, University of Bath), for her help in preparing material on radiopharmaceuticals.

References

1. *British Pharmaceutical Codex*. 10th edn. London: Pharmaceutical Press, 1973.
2. Breckenridge A. *The Report of a Working Party on the Addition of Drugs to Intravenous Infusion Fluids*. HC(76)9. London: DHSS, 1976.
3. Department of Health and Social Security. *Health Services Management: Manufacture of Products in the NHS*. HC(84)3. London: DHSS, 1984.
4. *Guidance to the NHS on the Licensing Requirements of the Medicines Act 1968*. London: Medicines Control Agency, 1992.
5. Specials MCA Guidance Note 14. *The Supply of Unlicensed Relevant Medicinal Products for Individual Patients*. London: Medicines Control Agency, 2000.
6. Risk Assessment of NHS Manufacturing. *Report of the Advisory Group on the Risk Assessment of Unlicensed Relevant Medicinal Products (Specials) within the NHS*. London: Department of Health, 2002.
7. Medicines Control Agency. *Rules and Guidance for Good Pharmaceutical Manufacture and Distribution*. London: The Stationery Office, 2002.
8. *British Pharmacopoeia*. London: The Stationery Office, 2001.
9. Audit conducted by Research and Development Team of UK National CIVAS Group 2001 (unpublished data).
10. Audit Commission. *A Spoonful of Sugar – Medicines Management in NHS Hospitals*. London: Audit Commission, 2001.
11. Farwell J. *Aseptic Dispensing for NHS Patients*. London: Department of Health, 1995.
12. Gandy R J, Beaumont I M, Lee M G, Cumming I. Risk management and the aseptic preparation of medicines. *Eur Hosp Pharm* 1998; 4: 114–119.
13. Plumridge R J, Sewell G J. Dose-banding of cytotoxic drugs: a new concept in cancer chemotherapy. *Am J Health-Systems Pharm* 2001; 58: 1760–1764.

14. Allwood M, Stanley A, Wright P, eds. *Cytotoxics Handbook*, 4th edn. Oxford: Radcliffe Medical Press, 2002.
15. Beaney A M. *Quality Assurance of Aseptic Preparation Services*, 3rd edn. London: Pharmaceutical Press, 2001.
16. Lee G M, Midcalf B. *Isolators for Pharmaceutical Applications*. London: HMSO, 1994.
17. MARC Guidelines. www.marcguidelines.com (accessed 19 November 2002).
18. Department of Health. *Guidance on Intrathecal Administration of Vinca Alkaloids*. London: Department of Health, 2001.
19. *Control of Substances Hazardous to Health Regulations*. London: Health and Safety Executive, 1994.

Further reading

Guild of Healthcare Pharmacists Compounding Interest Group. www.ghp.org.uk (accessed 19 November 2002).

Maltby P. The maze of regulations in radiopharmacy. *Hosp Pharm* 1999; 6: 42–45.

Management and Awareness of Risks of Cytotoxics (MARC) Programme. www.marcguidelines.com (accessed 20 August 2002).

Medicines Control Agency. *Rules and Guidance for Pharmaceutical Manufacturers and Distributors*. London: The Stationery Office, 1997.

National CIVAS Group. www.civas.co.uk (accessed 19 November 2002).

Needle R, Sizer T. *The CIVAS Handbook*. London: Pharmaceutical Press, 1998.

NHS Stability Database and UK Formulary of Extemporaneous Preparations. www.wpqa.co.uk (accessed 19 November 2002).

NHS Technical Specialist Education and Training (TSET). www.tset.org.uk (accessed 19 November 2002).

Palmer M. Radiopharmacy, the role of the pharmacist. *Hosp Pharm* 1999; 6: 38–41.

Pharmaceutical Isolator User Group. www.piug.org.uk (accessed 19 November 2002).

UK Radiopharmacy Group. www.ukrg.org.uk (accessed 19 November 2002).

5

Quality assurance

Ian M Beaumont

National Health Service (NHS) regional quality control (QC) laboratories were first established in 1966 following Health Memorandum HM(65)22 [1]. This dealt with the QC of purchased drugs and dressings, giving guidance to NHS regions on setting up regional QC services. The aim was to ensure that the quality of the products purchased through the regional purchasing system met a satisfactory standard. In the early 1970s the work of the laboratories was significantly extended following HSC(IS)128 *Application of the Medicines Act to Health Authorities*, which applied the principles of the Medicines Act to all pharmaceutical manufacturing operations undertaken by health authorities [2]. This required quality assurance (QA) and QC arrangements to be in place for all such activities and resulted in provision of QC laboratory facilities for each NHS manufacturing unit, located in most major pharmacy departments. It also resulted in them being subjected to regular inspection by the Medicines Inspectorate [3, 4].

In 1984, Health Circular HC(84)3 introduced a policy of costing hospital pharmaceutical manufacturing operations and required the NHS to engage in manufacture only if there was no satisfactory commercial source or if it was significantly more economical to do so [5]. This, along with the increasing commercial availability of hospital requirements, resulted in the rationalisation of both manufacturing and QC laboratory facilities through the remainder of the 1980s and the 1990s. Some NHS regions took the view that QA and QC services should be provided centrally at regional level, in order to make the best and most cost-effective use of the specialist staff and laboratory resources; this resulted in regional QC services based within one or two large laboratories on hospital sites within their region.

In recent years there has been (and continues to be) a very large increase in the number of pharmacy aseptic units preparing injections and other products, as well as an increase in the preparation of clinical trials materials. NHS Executive Letters EL(96)95 and EL(97)52 [6, 7] introduced requirements for regular internal and external quality audit of pharmacy aseptic preparation activities. The requirements established the role of the regional QA specialist in performing these external audits. These aseptic services, along with the remaining NHS manufacturing units, continue to require specialist QA and QC facilities as well as pharmacists and other QA staff with substantial skills and knowledge in QA, good pharmaceutical manufacturing practice, QC, audit, pharmaceutical sciences and technology, formulation and stability.

The NHS quality agenda and the role of the quality assurance pharmacist

Quality assurance

The assurance of quality in pharmaceutical products and services is of prime importance. Patients rely on pharmacists providing medicines which are consistently safe, efficacious and of suitable quality. Quality itself has a number of definitions – the *Concise Oxford Dictionary* defines quality as 'degree of excellence, relative nature or kind of character' [8]. This implies a rather subjective view of quality – comparative and difficult to quantify and measure. The total quality management (TQM) approach describes quality as 'meeting customer needs' [9]. TQM is a management philosophy which embraces all activities, through which the needs and expectations of the customer and the community are satisfied and through which the objectives of the organisation are met; these aims are achieved in the most cost-effective way by maximising the potential of all employees in a continuing drive for improvement. This is appropriate for pharmacy services, and aims to ensure that the service objectives are entirely organised around meeting customer needs.

A third approach to defining quality, and one which is most appropriate to be applied to pharmaceutical products, is the 'fitness for purpose' definition, as adopted in pharmaceutical manufacturing over many years. *The Rules and Guidance for Pharmaceutical Manufacturers and Distributors* (commonly called 'the Orange Guide' because of the colour of its cover) states that the quality objective in manufacturing is to ensure that the products are 'fit for their intended use' [10]. This definition can be applied in a quantitative sense, with quality parameters and limits being set against which all services or batches of products are tested and checked for compliance. Examples of this are product specifications comprising assays and service specifications comprising quantitative service parameters such as length of waiting times for prescriptions.

'Quality assurance' is the term applied to all the arrangements which influence the quality of the products or services supplied. The Orange Guide defines it as 'the sum total of the organised arrangements made with the object of ensuring that medicinal products are of the quality required for their intended use' [10]. In pharmaceutical manufacturing it encompasses both good manufacturing practice (GMP) and QC. GMP is the part of QA which ensures that products are consistently produced and controlled to the quality standards appropriate to their intended use. QC is the part of GMP concerned with sampling, specifications and testing, and with the release of products for use. Sharp provides a detailed discussion of these concepts in his text on quality in manufacture of health care products [11].

Clinical governance

A First Class Service: Quality in the New NHS introduced the concept of clinical governance to the NHS [12]. It defined the term as 'a framework through which NHS organisations are accountable for continuously improving the quality of their services and safeguarding high standards of care by creating an environment in which excellence in clinical care will flourish'. Chapter 9 of this book discusses the document and its impact on pharmacy. Pharmaceutical QA services have a long history of innovation and quality improvement of hospital pharmacy services at both local and national level. Many of the components of clinical governance have been well developed and in place for many years, for example, the issue of standards and guidance, QC and audit of manufacturing and aseptic services. Responsibility and accountability for quality of products prepared in licensed units have long been clearly placed with the quality controller. Quality improvement activities are a fundamental part of the QA pharmacist's role. Examples of this are audit, continuing professional development for QA and other pharmacy staff, the application of evidence-based good practice based on clear evidence provided through QC and monitoring data, and sound pharmaceutical research and development (R&D) work.

Risk management

Many aspects of pharmacy services have the potential to harm patients through errors or poor advice. Robust QA systems need to be in place to prevent this happening, especially for activities that carry the most risk. QA pharmacists have well-established systems for risk management of procurement activities and of licensed manufacturing and aseptic preparation services through systems of QC and audit, and plans are being developed nationally to extend this function across other high-risk areas of pharmacy.

Medication errors

In 2000 an expert group chaired by the Chief Medical Officer published a report entitled *An Organisation with a Memory* which summarised the scale and nature of serious failures in NHS health care and made recommendations on how lessons should be learnt from errors and near-misses and how to minimise the likelihood of repeating these errors in the future [13]. This was followed in 2001 by *Building a Safer NHS for Patients* [14], which set the NHS targets for implementing the recommendations from *An Organisation with a Memory* [13]. It established a new national agency, the National Patient Safety Agency, which has the remit of collecting and analysing information on adverse events in the NHS, assimilating other safety-related information, learning lessons and ensuring they are fed back into practice, producing solutions to prevent harm where risks are identified, specifying national goals and establishing mechanisms to track progress. Four specific risks were targeted for action by the NHS, two relating directly to pharmaceutical care. The first target was to reduce to zero by the end of 2001 the number of patients dying or being paralysed by maladministered spinal injections, and the second target was to reduce by 40% by 2005 the number of serious errors in the use of prescribed drugs.

QA pharmacists have a key contribution to make towards achieving these targets, in assisting with the reporting, analysis and feeding back of information regarding medication errors, and in ensuring that appropriate systems of QA, QC and audit are in place throughout all areas of pharmacy practice.

The aims of NHS pharmaceutical quality assurance services

The quality of medicines and their management are vital for the NHS. There are important health gains to be achieved from the use of quality-assured, clinically effective medicines. It is also important to manage the potential risks of using medicines which may be of an inappropriate quality and could result in poor efficacy and safety. As part of a team effort, the overall management of medicines requires specialist input from QA pharmacists and other QA staff. They can contribute an indepth knowledge of the pharmaceutical sciences, formulation and stability, QA systems and the total QC of medicines. The aims of pharmaceutical QA services are therefore assuring the quality of medicines and minimising the risk to NHS patients of receiving defective medicines. These aims are achieved by applying appropriate systems of QA, audit and QC to the purchasing and manufacturing/preparation of medicines in hospitals.

Pharmaceutical QA services include:

- development, issue, implementation and monitoring of standards and guidance relating to quality aspects of hospital pharmacy services and the management of medicines
- QA and QC of medicines purchased or manufactured/prepared for hospital patients
- quality audit of pharmacy technical services
- investigation and testing of defective medicines
- advisory services on all aspects of pharmaceutical QA and QC
- R&D, especially in the areas of pharmaceutical formulation and stability studies
- QC of medical gas installations in hospitals
- training of pharmacy staff
- laboratory and environmental testing services.

NHS QA services are coordinated nationally by the NHS Pharmaceutical Quality Control Committee, which includes regional QA pharmacists from throughout the UK. In addition to coordinating QA services the Committee also develops and issues policy, standards and guidance on a range of pharmaceutical QA issues. It operates a communications network at national and local levels, provides leadership and collective expert views, develops and promotes best practice and educational programmes and assists in maximising the efficient use of QA resources by sharing information. This information sharing includes the Analytical Information Centre (AIC) database containing summarised test data from all regional laboratories, and the UK Stability Database, which includes reports of stability studies carried out in QC laboratories across the UK. The Committee reports to the Chief Pharmacist at the Department of Health, and has close working relationships with pharmaceutical advisers, the Medicines Control Agency (MCA), Medical Devices Agency, Royal Pharmaceutical Society of Great Britain and other key national bodies and agencies.

Development, issue, implementation and monitoring of standards and guidance

QA staff are actively involved locally and nationally in the development of pharmaceutical technical standards and guidance for application to pharmacy services. The NHS Pharmaceutical Quality Control Committee has produced guidance documents covering a wide span of topics [15–18]. Implementation and monitoring of national and local standards/guidance are carried out on an ongoing basis through QC, environmental monitoring and audit programmes in hospital pharmacy manufacturing units and in both licensed and unlicensed aseptic dispensing units.

Quality assurance and quality control of medicines

Hospital manufacturing units

The manufacture of medicines is a complex operation and must conform to GMP requirements of the MCA [10]. These require a system of QA designed to build quality into each product at all stages of its manufacture. To this end, pharmaceutical QA services work closely with production staff and provide a series of checks, tests and controls throughout the manufacturing process as follows:

- microbiological and chemical testing where appropriate of ingredients, labels and packaging components, in-process samples and finished products
- checking and approval of all standard operating procedures and production documents
- environmental monitoring in clean and aseptic areas
- validating processes, equipment and procedures
- monitoring the performance of sterilisers
- pharmaceutical development work, including formulation development, stability studies and manufacturing and analytical method development and validation
- planned quality auditing at regular intervals
- liaison with the MCA.

Each manufacturing unit is required to be licensed under the Medicines Act, holding a manufacturer's specials licence. A requirement of the licence is that there must be a named production manager and named quality controller for the release for use of all products manufactured in the unit. This is a key role for QA pharmacists and other appropriately qualified and experienced QA staff. Before releasing each batch for use, the quality controller has to satisfy him-/herself that GMP, as laid down in MCA guidance, has been complied with, that all manufacturing and QC processes have been validated, that all checks and tests have been carried out and are satisfactory, that all documentation is satisfactory, and that all other factors which affect the product quality are satisfactory. This requires highly trained and competent QC staff who are fully aware of the quality, safety and efficacy requirements of pharmaceutical products.

Purchased medicines

Medicines are purchased by hospital pharmacists either through a system of regional contracts or through local purchasing arrangements with suppliers (see chapter 2). QA pharmacists have an important role in advising procurement staff on the quality and suitability of commercially manufactured pharmaceutical products purchased through the contracting system or purchased locally. Regional laboratories carry out work in assessing samples of products prior to contract awards. This can comprise laboratory testing for compliance with standards, and for bioequivalence where appropriate, and assessment of the packaging and labelling for correctness.

Unlicensed medicines are prepared by holders of manufacturers' specials licences or they may be imported from outside the UK. These products are frequently required for individual hospital patients with special needs when no suitable licensed equivalent is available.

Unlicensed medicines are not subject to the same controls as licensed medicines, and so special care needs to be taken during their purchase and use. The MCA and regional quality controllers have issued guidance on these issues [15, 19]. QA pharmacists have a key role in assessing and approving suppliers of specials, in evaluating and, if necessary, testing the products themselves before use. They can also make an important contribution in training and advising pharmacists and other users on risks associated with unlicensed medicines and the standards and controls to be applied.

Quality assurance of pharmacy services

Owing to their detailed knowledge and experience of the application of the principles of QA and GMP to manufacturing and aseptic dispensing activities, QA staff have developed their services in the last few years to encompass other areas of pharmacy services. A particular area is in extemporaneous dispensing activities. These carry a high risk to the patient if mistakes are made [20]. The risk of error can be reduced or eliminated by the application of appropriate QA and QC systems. QA pharmacists have, in some hospitals, introduced systems such as QC of dispensing ingredients, independent QC checking of documentation and testing and releasing of extemporaneously dispensed products. Further developments have included issuing guidance on standards, facilities and procedures for dispensing operations and the introduction of internal and external audit schemes. It is hoped that the application of quality systems to dispensing processes and other high-risk areas of pharmacy practice will become universal throughout pharmacy services in the near future.

Quality assurance of aseptic services

Aseptic preparation units in hospital pharmacies prepare a large range of injectable and other sterile products for individual patient use, including additives to infusion solutions, total parenteral nutrition (intravenous feeding) solutions, prefilled syringes and cytotoxic drug injections (see chapter 4). Many of these products have a narrow therapeutic range and carry a very high risk to the patient if they are not made up correctly or if they become contaminated with microorganisms [21]. There are many reports in the literature describing errors when injections have been made up by nursing or medical staff on the ward [22–30]. NHS guidance [31] states that, in order to minimise risks to patients, whenever possible these high-risk products should be prepared under pharmacy control in appropriate facilities; this was confirmed by the Audit Commission's advice in A *Spoonful of Sugar* [32]. As a result, there has been a large increase over the past decade in the activity of pharmacy aseptic units as high-risk aseptic preparation activities have been transferred to pharmacy control. Guidance on standards for aseptic services is given in the third edition of *Quality Assurance of Aseptic Preparation Services* [17]. This describes standards for facilities, procedures and controls to be applied, and also includes a useful chapter on the risks associated with aseptic preparation, and the management of these risks.

A priority for pharmaceutical QA services is working closely with these aseptic units to ensure the safety and quality of the products prepared. QA staff are routinely involved in assisting in the design of facilities, and in monitoring them using a series of regular environmental and personnel monitoring techniques (see later in this chapter). They are involved in training aseptic unit staff and regularly issue advice and guidance on all aspects of QA in aseptic preparation. They are also involved in quality audit processes (see below). In licensed units the QA officer is named as the quality controller, and has responsibility for releasing all products for use.

The continuing direct involvement of QA personnel with aseptic preparation activities will be a key future role for the QA service.

Quality audit

Quality audit is a systematic and independent examination to determine whether quality activities and related results comply with planned arrangements and whether these arrangements are implemented effectively and are suitable to achieve objectives [33].

QA pharmacists have been involved for many years in the application of audits to licensed manufacturing units and other pharmacy technical services such as radiopharmacy. In the 1990s aseptic dispensing in unlicensed units was the subject of two NHS Executive Letters, EL (96)95 and EL(97)52 [6, 7]. The former required hospitals to carry out an internal audit exercise and the latter set in place an ongoing system of external audits carried out by regional QA specialists every 12–18 months. These audits are now reported directly to the Chief Executives of NHS trusts and to the commissioners of these services, with areas requiring action highlighted. In 1999 the NHS Quality Control Committee issued a guidance booklet on quality audits and their application to hospital pharmacy technical services [18]. This describes audit processes and gives guidance on how they are applied in practice, along with a useful glossary of terms.

The audit system in pharmacy services is now firmly established as a key component of the NHS clinical governance agenda. Audit aims to improve quality continuously, assisting in the identification and management of risks and in the systems of learning from errors and near-misses described in recent NHS policy documents [13, 14].

Advisory services

The QA specialists' knowledge of quality systems, pharmaceutical QA, audit and QC is utilised widely for advising pharmacists, other health care professionals, the NHS Executive, health authorities, NHS trusts and primary care trusts.

Research and development

R&D plays an active part in the role of the pharmaceutical QA specialist. As clinical practice changes there is a constant need for the development of new formulations and for determining their shelf-lives. R&D activity is therefore mainly focused around formulation and pharmaceutical development projects and stability studies, although much other R&D work around analytical method development and validation, method transfer, bioavailability and compatibility with packaging components is carried out.

There is a particularly heavy demand for R&D activities associated with aseptic preparation of medicines, often involving complex mixtures of drug substances and drug-packaging component interaction.

Dedicated laboratory and controlled temperature and humidity storage facilities for both real-time and accelerated stability studies are usually available in the larger laboratories and regional QC centres. Data from stability studies performed in UK hospitals are summarised in the *UK Stability Database* [34].

Testing piped medical gas installations

Standards for medical gas installations in hospitals are laid down in a Health Technical Memorandum (HTM2022) [35]. This covers the design, installation, validation, verification and maintenance of pipeline systems. Medical gases are classified as medicinal products under the Medicines Act, and the quality controller has responsibility for the QC of the medical gases supplied by the pipeline system.

QA personnel are regularly required to visit operating theatres, wards and other clinical areas where medical gas pipelines are used, to carry out testing of the identity, quality and purity of the gases prior to them being taken into use [36]. The tests involve using portable equipment including paramagnetic oxygen analysers, infrared gas analysers, particle filter test units and chemical reagent tubes. A permit-to-work system is used for recording details of work performed.

QA staff are also involved in advising on suitable procedures for the handling, storage and control of medical gases.

Training of pharmacy staff

QA staff are regularly involved in the provision of training on a wide range of QA issues to preregistration pharmacists and to other pharmacy personnel.

Defective medicines

Great care is taken to ensure that all medicines used in hospitals are of a suitable quality. However, occasionally defects are identified in medicinal products: this requires rapid and reliable action to determine the severity of the defect and its implications to the patient and to other patients who may be receiving treatment from the affected batch.

Defects may be reported by patients themselves, or from any health care professional. They may be relatively minor in nature, for example chipped tablets, or potentially very serious, for example suspected contamination of an intravenous injection. Systems are in place in all hospitals to communicate rapidly the details of the defect, and if appropriate to take the sample to the regional QC laboratory for investigation.

In the laboratory, rapid response procedures are then initiated to investigate the defect, carry out laboratory testing if necessary, and to communicate the outcome of the investigation as appropriate. Serious defects are reported directly to the Defective Medicines Reporting Centre at the MCA and, if it is considered necessary, a formal drug alert is sent to regional QC laboratories to be communicated throughout the NHS [37]. In serious cases the affected batches are withdrawn from use.

Laboratory services

QC laboratory facilities can be divided into two specialist areas: pharmaceutical chemistry and microbiology.

Pharmaceutical chemistry facilities comprise areas for classical 'wet' chemical methods of analysis and gravimetric analysis, along with laboratory areas for a range of physical testing methods such as melting point, hardness, friability, disintegration and dissolution testing. Wet analysis includes aqueous and non-aqueous volumetric analysis (although the use of burettes has now largely been taken over by the use of computer-controlled autotitrator systems). Other chemistry laboratory areas are dedicated to instrumental methods of analysis, such as spectrophotometry (ultraviolet/visible, Fourier transform infrared and atomic absorption), polarimetry, refractometry, subvisual liquid particle counting and chromotography (thin-layer, gas and high-performance liquid chromatography). The use of high-performance liquid chromatography in pharmaceutical analysis has grown enormously over recent years owing to the ability of this technique to separate and quantify mixtures of components in aqueous formulations. It is also utilised very heavily in pharmaceutical development and in stability studies since it can be used to separate and quantify active drugs and degradation products produced on storage.

Analytical methods used in the laboratories are primarily pharmacopoeial, taken from the *British Pharmacopoeia* or *European Pharmacopoeia* or from other international pharmacopoeias as appropriate. However in many cases no suitable official monograph exists, so in-house specifications are developed and validated. The frequent changes in and development of new clinical treatments require the formulation and QC testing of new products, the ongoing development of new product specifications and analytical methods. This presents a variety of interesting challenges to laboratory staff, requiring a high level of scientific knowledge and the ability to apply it to new problems.

Samples entering the laboratory are many and varied, ranging from pharmacopoeial raw materials, in-process samples and finished products from hospital manufacturing units to samples of unlicensed medicines. These may have been purchased by hospitals from commercial holders of manufacturers' specials licences or may have been imported from anywhere in the world to meet a specific patient's need. Samples may also be of any licensed medicinal product being assessed for its suitability for purchase, or may be the subject of a defective medicines report, referred to the laboratory for investigation. In many cases (such as in the case of suspected defective medicines) the analysis and assessment of the product are required urgently. It is therefore essential that suitable laboratory resources and expertise are available to deal with these when required.

A key area of work of the laboratories is R&D covering a range of activities including new product formulation and pharmaceutical development, analytical method development and validation, and stability studies. In many laboratories this work runs alongside other QC work with the same staff carrying out QC testing and R&D activities, but in some larger regional laboratories a separate R&D section with its own dedicated laboratories is in place. These dedicated R&D laboratories are mainly equipped with chromatographic equipment, especially high-specification computer-controlled high-performance liquid chromatography equipment utilising diode array, fluorimetric, refractive index and other detectors, along with gradient elution programmers and autoinjectors allowing the equipment to be utilised 24 hours a day. Data generated are analysed by sophisticated multichannel data-handling systems. In the north-west NHS region's R&D laboratory, for instance, there are currently such systems in constant use.

As a result of the wide variety of samples submitted for QC testing, along with the involvement in R&D activities, laboratory staff obtain a large breadth of experience in pharmaceutical analysis. As well as pharmacists, other laboratory staff are trained to graduate or higher level in chemistry, microbiology or an associated science. Opportunities exist for continuing professional development and many QC laboratory staff have undertaken external courses such as the MSc in Pharmaceutical Technology and Quality Assurance, run jointly by the NHS and Leeds University.

Pharmaceutical microbiology facilities comprise areas for carrying out a wide range of microbiological tests on pharmaceuticals and raw materials such as total viable counts, incubation and reading of settle plates (and media from other environmental and personnel-monitoring techniques such as active air sampling, surface testing or finger dabs), organism identification, preservative efficacy testing and microbiological stability studies. There are also dedicated areas for carrying out endotoxin testing (using automated *Limulus* amoebocyte lysate) and dedicated aseptic facilities for sterility testing.

The quantity of work passing through the pharmaceutical microbiology laboratory has increased enormously over recent years, reflecting the large increase in activity of hospital pharmacy aseptic preparation and dispensing units and the publication of standards laying down high levels of monitoring [17]. Each aseptic unit is required to undertake a programme of sessional, daily, weekly and quarterly validation and monitoring tests, which results in large numbers of settle plates and other microbiological media, along with samples of finished products for sterility testing or endotoxin testing. Microbiology laboratory facilities have therefore increased in size through the 1990s in response to this increasing demand.

A key element of the work of the pharmaceutical microbiologist is the interpretation of the significance of the results obtained from the various tests performed and their effect on the quality and safety of aseptically prepared and manufactured products. This requires a constant awareness of trends in results for each aseptic unit, and the ability to react quickly and issue advice and guidance to the pharmacist supervising aseptic preparation if problems are found. Modern Laboratory Information Management Systems (LIMS) utilising bar-coding and direct data entry by laboratory staff, coupled with automatic trend analysis and electronic reporting to the aseptic or manufacturing unit, facilitate these processes.

The standard of laboratory work performed is of prime importance in all hospital QC laboratories. All results generated are relied upon by QA and other pharmacists in making critically important decisions regarding release of batches of medicines for use in patients, and so it is essential that all results are valid. Quality systems are in place to ensure this is the case, including systems for staff training, supervision and checking, method validation, calibration, traceability of standards, documentation, internal QC procedures and participation in interlaboratory testing schemes. The NHS Pharmaceutical Interlaboratory Testing Scheme (PITS) has run successfully in this regard over the last 20 years, with over 40 hospital QC laboratories participating. Many laboratories follow an ISO 9000, quality system model [38, 39]. Some laboratories are accredited by UKAS, the United Kingdom Accreditation Service for compliance with ISO/IEC 17025 standards [40]. All laboratories associated with licensed manufacturing operations are subject to regular (biennial) inspection by the MCA inspectors. The small number of laboratories associated with hospital units producing CE-marked medical devices are also subject to Notified Body inspection.

Environmental monitoring services

Specialist QC staff are involved in the monitoring of hospital pharmacy clean and aseptic environments used for the manufacture and aseptic dispensing of medicines, along with other hospital clean areas such as ultraclean ventilation systems in operating theatres, clean isolation rooms in bone marrow units and hospital sterilising and disinfecting units (HSDUs). Portable monitoring equipment consisting of a range of physical and microbiological equipment is used.

Physical testing has several components: first, airborne subvisual particle counting, using laser-equipped particle counters capable of counting particles as small as 0.3 μm. A second aspect is air velocity measurements using anemometers for calculating the rate of air exchange in clean rooms and for ensuring that devices such as laminar air flow cabinets and pharmaceutical isolators are operating within the required parameters. Air pressure differential monitoring between different categories of clean rooms is undertaken using portable manometers. Filter integrity testing is carried out using dispersed oil particle generators and photometric detection equipment to ensure that high-efficiency particulate air (HEPA) filters and their housings are not leaking. Finally, operator protection testing is carried out using potassium iodide discus equipment.

Microbiological monitoring comprises settle plate testing, active air sampling, surface swabbing, finger dabs and other techniques designed to monitor levels of environmental microorganisms in the clean/aseptic area and to demonstrate whether acceptable levels are exceeded.

Owing to the specialised nature of this work, and the high cost of some of the test equipment, these services are often organised on a regional or group of hospitals basis.

The future

Because of its historical background, QC services have mainly focused on laboratory services and the provision of QA, QC and audit to technical areas of hospital pharmacy practice. All of these will remain important. Set against the NHS clinical governance agenda and the need to ensure high-quality pharmacy services are designed around the patient, the intention for the future is to widen the focus to encompass the QA aspects of pharmacy services in general. This will build on the considerable strengths of the service in terms of its expertise in the areas of QA, quality improvements, audit and risk management.

In line with *The NHS Plan* [41] and *Pharmacy in the Future* [42], QA services will continue to develop to play an increasing role in assuring the quality of pharmaceutical services and products for patients, especially in the development of more comprehensive systems for management of risks, and for learning from and preventing errors. There will be a greater input into assuring the quality of high-risk activities such as preparation and handling of aseptic products, clinical trials materials and unlicensed medicines, and increasing challenges in ensuring that appropriate QA arrangements are developed for the products of new technologies, such as gene therapy products and a rapidly increasing number of monoclonal antibody products.

The present national network of QA staff, led by the NHS Pharmaceutical Quality Control Committee, is important in ensuring the coordination of laboratory work, elimination of duplication, unification of standards across the NHS and the dissemination of information. This will continue to develop. There will be a move towards extending services into the primary care sector, in particular to developing and applying standards, auditing procedures for dispensing and giving access to the QA pharmacists' information and expertise on quality of medicines.

In the NHS of the future, in which a comprehensive range of services is provided to meet the needs of individual patients, and where quality will be continuously improved and errors minimised, the QA pharmacist and NHS Pharmaceutical Quality Control Service will have a key role in delivering these objectives.

References

1.   Ministry of Health. *National Health Service. Quality Control of Hospital Supplies of Drugs and Dressings.* HM(65)22. London: Ministry of Health, 1965.
2.   Department of Health and Social Security. *Application of the Medicines Act to Health Authorities.* Health Service Circular (Interim Series) HSC(IS)128. London: Department of Health, 1975.
3.   Sprake J M. The development of quality assurance in the Trent region, England. *J Clin Pharm* 1977; 2: 17–21.
4.   Sprake J M. An increasingly attractive specialty. *Pharm J* 1980; 224: 600–601.
5.   Department of Health and Social Security. *Health Services Management: Manufacture of Products in the NHS.* HC(84)3. London: DHSS, 1984.
6.   Department of Health. *Aseptic Dispensing for NHS Patients.* Executive Letter EL(96)95. London: Department of Health, 1996.
7.   Department of Health. *Aseptic Dispensing for NHS Patients.* Executive Letter EL(97)52. London: Department of Health, 1997.
8.   *Concise Oxford Dictionary.* Oxford: Oxford University Press, 1986.
9.   BS7850-1: 1994. ISO 9004-4: 1993. *Total Quality Management. Guidelines for Quality Improvement.* London: British Standards Institution.
10. Medicines Control Agency. *Rules and Guidance for Pharmaceutical Manufacturers and Distributors.* London: The Stationery Office, 2002.
11. Sharp J. *Quality in the Manufacture of Medicines and other Healthcare Products.* London: Pharmaceutical Press, 2000.
12. Department of Health. *A First Class Service: Quality in the New NHS.* London: The Stationery Office, 1998.
13. Department of Health. *An Organisation with a Memory – Report of an Expert Group on Learning from Adverse Events in the NHS Chaired by the Chief Medical Officer.* London: Department of Health, 2000.
14. Department of Health. *Building a Safer NHS for Patients. Implementing an Organisation with a Memory.* London: Department of Health, 2001.
15. NHS Pharmaceutical Quality Control Committee. *Guidance for the Purchase and Supply of Unlicensed Medicinal Products. Notes for Prescribers and Pharmacists,* 2nd edn. Liverpool: Quality Control Committee, 2001.
16. Lee M G, Midcalf B. *Isolators for Pharmaceutical Applications.* London: HMSO, 1994.
17. Beaney A M. *Quality Assurance of Aseptic Preparation Services,* 3rd edn. London: Pharmaceutical Press, 2001.
18. NHS Pharmaceutical Quality Control Committee. *Quality Audits and their Application to Hospital Pharmacy Technical Services.* Liverpool: Quality Control Committee, 1999.
19. Medicines Control Agency. *Guidance Note No. 14. The Supply of Unlicensed Relevant Medicinal Products for Individual Patients.* London: Medicines Control Agency, 2000.

20. Anonymous. Boots pharmacist and trainee cleared of baby's manslaughter, but fined for dispensing a defective medicine. *Pharm J* 2000; 264: 390–392.

21. Anonymous. Two children die after receiving infected TPN solutions. *Pharm J* 1994; 252: 596.

22. Ernot L, Thoren S, Sandell E. Studies on microbial contamination of infusion fluids arising from drug additions and administration. *Pharm Suec* 1973; 10: 141–146.

23. Cos G E. Bacterial contamination of drip sets. *NZ Med J* 1973; 77: 390–391.

24. Woodside W, Woodside W M, D'Arcy E M, Pate R W. Intravenous infusions as vehicles for infection. *Pharm J* 1975; 215: 606.

25. Deeks E N, Natsios G A. Contamination of infusion fluids by bacteria and fungi during preparation and administration. *Am J Hosp Pharm* 1971; 28: 764–767.

26. D'Arcy P F, Woodside M E. Drug additives, a potential source of bacterial contamination of infusion fluids. *Lancet* 1973; ii: 96.

27. Quercia R A, Hiels S W, Klimek J J *et al.* Bacteriologic contamination of intravenous infusion delivery systems in an intensive care unit. *Am J Med* 1986; 80: 364–368.

28. O'Hare M C B, Bradley A M, Gallagher T, Shields M D. Errors in administration of intravenous drugs (letter). *BMJ* 1995; 310: 1536–1537.

29. Cousins D H, Upton D R. Medication error 125: parenteral vial errors must stop. *Pharm Pract* 1999; 9: 220–221.

30. Cousins D H, Upton D R. Medication error 62: act now to prevent KCl deaths. *Pharm Pract* 1996; 6: 307–310.

31. Department of Health. *Controls Assurance Standards: Medicines Management (Safe and Secure Handling): Criterion 5 – Unlicensed Aseptic Dispensing.* London: Department of Health, 2001.

32. Audit Commission. *A Spoonful of Sugar – Medicines Management in NHS Hospitals.* London: Audit Commission, 2001.

33. ISO 10011–1. *1990 Guide to Quality Systems Auditing. Part 1: Auditing.* Geneva: International Standards Organisation, 1990.

34. Grassby P F. *UK NHS Stability Database.* Penarth: St Mary's Pharmaceutical Unit, 2002.

35. *NHS Estates.* Health Technical Memorandum HTM2022. London: HMSO, 1994.

36. O'Sullivan J, Beaumont I M. Piped medical gas testing – the new HTM 2022. *Hosp Pharm* 1994; 1: 94–96.

37. Medicines Control Agency. *Defective Medicinal Products: Guidance on Reporting Accidents with, and Defects in, Medicinal Products.* London: Department of Health, 1999.

38. BS EN ISO 9000. *Quality Management Systems. Fundamentals and Vocabulary.* London: British Standards Institution, 2000.

39. BS EN ISO 9001. *Quality Management Systems. Requirements.* London: British Standards Institution, 2001.

40. BS EN ISO/IEC 17025. *General Requirements for the Competence of Testing and Calibration Laboratories.* London: British Standards Institution, 2000.

41. Department of Health. *The NHS Plan.* London: The Stationery Office, 2000.

42. Department of Health. *Pharmacy in the Future*. London: Department of Health, 2000.

Further reading

Beaney A M. *Quality Assurance of Aseptic Preparation Services*, 3rd edn. London: Pharmaceutical Press, 2001.

Medicines Control Agency. *Rules and Guidance for Pharmaceutical Manufacturers and Distributors*. London: The Stationery Office, 2002.

Sharp J. *Quality in the Manufacture of Medicines and other Healthcare Products*. London: Pharmaceutical Press, 2000.

6

Medicines information

Peter Golightly

Medicines information (MI) has developed as a speciality of hospital pharmacy within the UK National Health Service (NHS), and is mirrored by similar service developments in advanced health care systems in most of the developed world, including Europe, the USA and Australasia. The models adopted, however, vary according to the health systems and practices in a particular country, and the main influences, opportunities and practices that define a national health care model. Although most MI services are provided by pharmacists as part of the portfolio of services provided by a hospital pharmacy service, there are models where doctors, nurses and other technical staff have a more predominant role in the provision of such services than is the practice in the UK.

History

The history and structure of MI services in the UK largely reflect those of the NHS in which it functions, and to which most of its activities are directed. Through the 1960s hospital pharmacy was undergoing a radical change, especially with the development of ward-based, patient-focused activities – clinical pharmacy. The pharmacist's traditional role of compounding, dispensing and medicines supply was being replaced by the provision of prescribing and clinical support through clinical advice to doctors and nurses, and information provision direct to patients. The hospital pharmacist became the ward-based expert on drugs and therapeutics. However, this huge expansion of activity was accompanied by a parallel demand for high-quality and reliable information to support these activities. Prior to this, information on medicines had been acquired either from personal knowledge or from standard reference sources, such as formularies, pharmacopoeias and textbooks, traditionally supplied by pharmacists. The requirement for information and advisory support to health care professionals with a medicines-related role was further supported by a number of simultaneous developments. The so-called 'therapeutic explosion' in the 1960s and 1970s made available a vast array of new and potent drugs with both increased efficacy and toxicity. These rapidly replaced the more traditionally compounded medicines. Accompanying this was an 'information explosion' in which the availability of published, critically assessed, clinical information and evidence increased dramatically. This literature covered all aspects of drugs, including their pharmacology, pharmacokinetics, comparative clinical efficacy, toxicity, use in specific circumstances such as pregnancy and the pharmaceutics of formulation and drug delivery. It is estimated that there are currently over 12 000 medical and pharmaceutical journals worldwide, the majority of which have the potential to include information on drugs. The establishment of these new roles for hospital pharmacists, including MI services, was formalised in the Noel Hall Report [1].

The demand for high-quality, commercially independent, evaluated, rapid and patient-oriented information from all members of the health care team led to the development of Drug Information Services, recently renamed Medicines Information Services to reflect current terminology and practice.

Structure and activities

The first MI services in the UK were established at the London Hospital and Leeds General Infirmary in 1969 [2, 3] followed over the next 10 years by a UK-wide network of local and regional services. This was supported by recommendations from a working party of the Pharmaceutical Society of Great Britain [4]. Local MI centres have been established in about 270 mainly acute hospitals, largely providing a service to their base hospital and associated local health care community. Twenty regional MI centres, including national centres in Wales and Northern Ireland, and four regional centres in Scotland have subsequently been reduced to 15 through a series of NHS reorganisations. These services have been brought together in a structured and coordinated national network (UK Medicines Information – UKMI), to which both local and regional services contribute skills, expertise, knowledge and resources. The network is coordinated and provided with strategic leadership by a national representative body, the UK Medicines Information Pharmacists Group (UKMIPG).

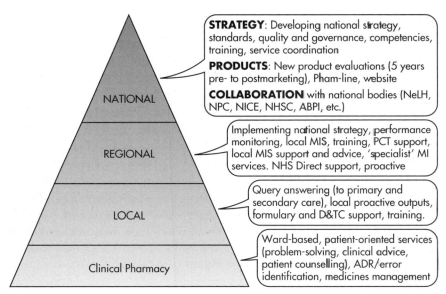

Figure 6.1 Structure of medicines information (MI) services in the UK. NeLH, National Electronic Library for Health; NPC, National Prescribing Centre; NICE, National Institute for Clinical Excellence; NHSC, National Horizon Scanning Centre; ABPI, Association of the British Pharmaceutical Industry; MIS, medicines information service; PCT, primary care trust; D&TC, drugs and therapeutics committees; ADR, adverse drug reaction.

MI services in the UK have therefore developed on a pyramidal tiered basis, creating a network structure that allows provision of services and support at all levels of health care, whilst being mutually supportive, cost-effective and responsive to its users. Each level of the pyramid acts as a back-up to the level below, but also contributes to the level above. Each level undertakes a range of activities that is most appropriate to the users of the service, produces maximum benefit of scale and reduces duplication, both at and between the same operational levels (Figure 6.1). The development of these services has been well described and supported in the professional literature and recognised by government and other official organisations [5–13].

Aims and strategy

The aims of the MI service are to facilitate high-quality patient care, through the promotion of the safe, effective and economic use of medicines, by the provision of accurate, timely, appropriate, evidence-based and unbiased information and advice on all aspects relating to the use of medicines. These have been the core principles that have formed the framework of the service since its inception. It is largely through the demonstration of the fulfilment of these aims that the service has achieved its current high level of use, acceptability and recognition amongst its users and in the broader NHS.

In order to achieve and maintain the level and quality of service that these aims demand, a range of core principles have been developed which underpin all the activities of the service. These state that MI services will:

- apply evidence-based principles in the provision of impartial, evaluated, accurate and timely information. This will be in a suitable format, that is, pertinent to the user's needs and readily understood
- provide professional advice to support and influence clinical decisions with respect to patient care and to enable the individual to make a balanced choice
- keep abreast of developments in therapeutics, professional practice, technology and information sources to support continuing professional development within the speciality and to ensure that the service provided is as up-to-date as possible
- be readily accessible and responsive to user needs
- network with others to share information and experience at local, regional and national levels.

NHS changes have given opportunities to develop MI; there have also been increased demands on the MI service. In light of this, a 5-year UK-wide strategy, *Better Information for Managing Medicines*, was produced in 2000, to establish a framework for the provision and development of the service up to the year 2005 [13]. The strategy gained the approval and endorsement of the national health departments of the four UK countries and is being implemented widely at all levels of the service. Three 'strategic aims' identified are:

- Extend the service available to primary care
- Develop the service in secondary care
- Provide support at national level.

Some of the main drivers for the development of the service through this strategy include the development of primary care trusts as the lead for health care provision and commissioning, the introduction of NHS Direct in England and Wales and NHS24 in Scotland, the arrival of new prescribers (nurses, pharmacists and others), the provision of nationally driven guidance from the National Institute for Clinical Excellence (NICE) and the general desire to manage new drug entry. The development of information technology (IT) initiatives, such as the internet and the National Electronic Library for Health (NeLH), also influence the MI agenda, as they make information on medicines directly available to health professionals and the public.

Roles and skills

MI pharmacists undertake a wide range of roles and activities which encompass provision of information and advice on all aspects of medicines, including safety, prescribing, administration, pharmaceutics and availability. These roles are applied at both a clinical level to facilitate individual patient care, and at a strategic level to facilitate decision-making processes in the production of medicines-related policies, the rational introduction and use of medicines (new and established) in the NHS and the production of guidelines and other tools to ensure the appropriate, safe and cost-effective use of medicines. The MI pharmacist therefore has to have the knowledge and skills to undertake these roles in an effective manner. These skills fall into a number of broad categories, as shown in Table 6.1, and are the basis for a person specification for an MI pharmacist. However, this portfolio of skills is not unique to an MI pharmacist; many will be possessed by effective and experienced clinical pharmacists, further illustrating that the origins of MI are firmly rooted in clinical pharmacy. Indeed, an effective MI pharmacist has to be, first and foremost, a competent clinical pharmacist with an indepth knowledge of therapeutics and its processes, and should, where possible, continue to provide a local clinical pharmacy role to facilitate an appropriate knowledge level and the ability to make the outputs of the MI service clinically and patient-relevant. The MI pharmacist will then have to develop the other skills outlined and, in some cases, to a higher level, in order to undertake the additional roles of an MI pharmacist. The training and competencies required to achieve and maintain these skills are discussed later.

Ethics and legal issues

All pharmacists should be aware of the legal and ethical principles governing the practice of the profession. MI, as a specialised function, has no UK case law, as far as is known, relating to the provision of the service by hospital pharmacists. The whole pharmacy profession is governed by the legal and ethical principles set out by its own regulatory body, and published in *Medicines, Ethics and Practice – A Guide for Pharmacists* [14]. Although it contains no specific reference to the

Table 6.1 Skill requirements for a medicines information pharmacist

Skill	Scope
Clinical	Knowledge and understanding of all aspects of drugs, therapeutic processes and procedures, disease pathology and management
Communication	Verbal: interrogating enquirers, determining the enquiry, obtaining appropriate and adequate background information, giving verbal responses, telephone techniques Written: writing reports, enquiry replies, bulletins; writing to the level of the recipient; converting data into concise and usable outputs; use of 'plain English'
Critical appraisal	Critically appraise and assess clinical and pharmaceutical literature, content and quality of commercial claims for medicines; working knowledge of medical statistics, including appropriateness and limitations; construction of clinical trials; pharmacoeconomics
Information management	Resource utilisation, e.g. searching primary literature (Medline, Embase, etc.), databases, internet, in-house and library resources; interpreting data retrieved; determining cost-effective and quality resources; systems design for in-house storage and retrieval of data
Interpersonal	Ability to work on own initiative; to prioritise work, self-assess performance and work quality and manage time effectively
Information technology (IT)	Ability to use IT resources for acquiring and disseminating information and service outputs. Understanding applications of IT. Keyboard skills
Management	Manage resources and people
Training	Ability to train pharmacists and other professionals requiring these skills or knowledge, e.g. preregistration pharmacists, pharmacists, nurses, doctors, etc.

practice of MI, the section 'Code of Ethics and Standards' does include statements which have direct applicability to the service:

- acting in the interests of patients and the public
- keeping up-to-date
- maintaining confidentiality
- getting the right level of information to patients.

Specifically regarding information provision, the guide states:

> Pharmacists and staff providing information and advice on health related issues must have an adequate level of current knowledge and information about relevant subjects; ensure that all advice is independent and not compromised by commercial considerations; seek appropriate and sufficient information from the enquirer to enable them to provide informed advice; and continually review their knowledge and keep up to date regarding new products.

From these statements it can be seen that MI pharmacists not only have a duty to fulfil certain obligations in providing their own professional service, but also have a role in facilitating other pharmacists in meeting their professional obligations. MI pharmacists are also a source of advice on legal and ethical issues routinely confronting all pharmacists, as well as on all legal and ethical issues relating to the prescribing, supply and administration of medicines by other health care professions.

UKDIPG (now UKMIPG) has published guidelines which cover the legal and ethical issues confronting MI pharmacists in the course of their duties [15]. These are, again, issues that will need to be considered by all pharmacists, but which have a more immediate significance to an MI pharmacist. The main issues are identified in Table 6.2.

Table 6.2 Legal and ethical issues in medicines information

Issue	Details
Negligence and liability	A medicines information (MI) pharmacist has a duty to ensure that all information and advice supplied is as accurate and comprehensive as could reasonably be expected. If that information or advice, when acted on, causes loss or damage to a patient, the MI pharmacist may be liable in negligence. For the MI pharmacist to be shown to be negligent it must be established that the MI pharmacist had a duty of care towards the patient, that the duty of care was breached and that damage to the patient occurred. It is, therefore, incumbent on an MI pharmacist to keep up-to-date as far as is reasonable with current developments and knowledge, to use all reasonably available resources to provide the information required, to present that information in a usable and intelligible form and to act in a professional manner which is appropriate to the skills possessed and the service offered by an MI pharmacist. Working to defined standards with agreed minimum resources and complying with standards for safe systems of work and documentation are part of this process.

(continued)

Table 6.2 *Continued*

Issue	*Details*
Unlicensed and clinical trial medicines	MI pharmacists can provide information and advice about unlicensed medicines or unlicensed uses of medicines as long as the enquirer or user is clearly informed that this is the case.
Proactive information	The same principles apply to written proactive information, for example, that supplied in bulletins or new-product evaluations. MI pharmacists should be able to demonstrate the process undertaken to produce the information. Disclaimers, although bringing to the attention of the information users their responsibilities in using that information, do not negate the liability of the MI pharmacist supplying the information. These issues apply to both hard-copy and electronically published information.
Defamation	MI pharmacists have a duty when providing information to ensure that information is accurate, fair and produced from demonstrable and quality evidence. Failure to do so, leading to unreasonable loss of commercial success of a medicine, could lead to the pursuance of 'defamation of product' by a pharmaceutical company. However, a genuine error or omission would not normally be grounds for such an action.
Confidentiality	MI pharmacists are bound by all aspects of patient and commercial confidentiality. For patients, any information about individual patients gained through the processes of enquiry handling, e.g. obtaining adequate background information to tailor a response, is covered by the rules of confidentiality, and should not be disclosed to a third party, except in certain exceptional, defined situations, e.g. if the patient's safety is at risk. This duty of confidentiality also applies to more difficult situations of potential disclose, such as to the police or to parents of patients. Confidentiality of commercially sensitive information, supplied by a pharmaceutical company to an MI pharmacist, is also an important issue. Information that is not in the public domain and which could be considered to be of commercial interest to a third party, e.g. another company, must be considered commercially confidential and only disclosed if the source from which the information was originally obtained gives explicit approval.

(continued)

Table 6.2   *Continued*

Issue	*Details*
Copyright	MI pharmacists must comply with the requirements of the current copyright legislation. They have a high requirement for acquiring, storing and distributing copies of published information which has to take account of the requirements of the legislation.
Data protection	MI pharmacists must comply with the requirements of current data protection legislation when keeping records of personal details of patients or enquirers, for whatever purposes.
Information to special users	From time to time, MI pharmacists may be requested to supply information to non-health care enquirers concerning medicines-related issues. These may include the police, coroners and legal representatives (when the MI pharmacist may be expected to be an expert witness) and the media (for publication or use in the lay press). In all situations the MI pharmacist will act only after determination of and in accordance with local policies and procedures, which may mean referring the enquirer to a more appropriate source for dealing with a particular issue.

The legal and ethical framework within which MI pharmacists provide the MI service is defined by both that of the profession of pharmacy and its own Code of Practice for Medicines Information Pharmacists [14, 15].

Clinical governance and risk management

The concept of clinical governance was introduced into the NHS by *A First Class Service: Quality in the New NHS* [16]. Chapter 9 will discuss clinical governance further, but clinical governance is an important part of the current MI agenda. In September 1999, the Royal Pharmaceutical Society published a framework for clinical governance in pharmacy [17]. Four principal components are identified for achieving excellence in practice:

1. Clear lines of responsibility and accountability for overall quality of clinical care
2. A comprehensive programme of quality improvement activities (e.g. audit, continuing professional development, research and development)
3. Clear policies aimed at managing risks
4. Procedures for identification of poor performance.

MI services in the UK, through UKMIPG, are committed to developing clinical governance programmes for the service and a national infrastructure has been developed to facilitate the development and implementation of a comprehensive programme, including guidelines on the role of clinical governance in MI services [18]. Clinical governance in MI has a number of components; success in all components is essential for the delivery of a high-quality service. The tools used for clinical governance in MI are those applicable to any area of health care provision. Those developed specifically within MI include:

- standards and quality assurance
- audit programmes
- user satisfaction surveys
- benchmarking schemes
- evidence-based practice
- continuing professional development
- training programmes
- risk assessment/management schemes
- appraisal schemes
- sharing best practice.

The first national standards for MI services were introduced in 1990 and have undergone several revisions and expansions in the last decade. The standards relate to the core activity of MI services – enquiry answering, including a standard for the minimum resources that a local MI service would be expected to have available in order to undertake enquiry answering effectively. The achievement of the standard in this activity area requires the availability of appropriate and trained staff, a definable communication infrastructure, quantifiable and consistent criteria to measure user satisfaction of the service, and quantifiable criteria for assessing the quality of enquiry answers. The four principal elements within this are:

1. Documentation of the complete enquiry process
2. Analysis of the enquiry
3. Utilisation and interpretation of appropriate resources
4. Construction and delivery of an appropriate, timely and evidence-based answer.

and for each element the enquiry is further classified into one of three levels of complexity. A straightforward enquiry requiring use of simple information resources with little interpretation of the information (for example, tablet identification) will require a different level of assessment than a complex clinical enquiry requiring use of multiple resources, interpretation of the evidence and construction of an answer tailored to a specific patient.

The second set of standards to be developed relate to proactive activities, such as bulletin production, which includes elements of text production, proof-reading and accuracy checking, and adherence to legal requirements such as copyright.

The third set of standards relate to continuing education and training and are defined according to the level of experience and responsibility that the pharmacist has within the MI service.

Additional elements of clinical governance implementation in MI include critical incident/'near-miss' reporting schemes, dialogue with principal stakeholders and involvement with commissioning of specialist services.

MI services have a dual role in clinical governance: internal and external.

Internal

MI pharmacists individually and the MI network as a whole must accept responsibility for provision of a high-quality service which meets the needs of its users. This can be achieved by formulation and adoption of clinical governance action plans incorporating the elements outlined in the section above.

External

In addition to improving their own performance, MI pharmacists are well placed to contribute to a wider clinical governance agenda within the NHS by supporting with evidence-based data:

- hospital clinical pharmacy services
- formularies
- medicines management programmes
- prescribing advice
- drug and therapeutics committees/area prescribing committees
- local formulation of clinical guidelines/protocols
- dissemination of good practice
- input to audit programmes and quality initiatives
- training and continuing professional development programmes
- shared-care support.

The framework developed in the UK for achieving quality within MI services through implementing an appropriate clinical governance process is outlined in Figure 6.2.

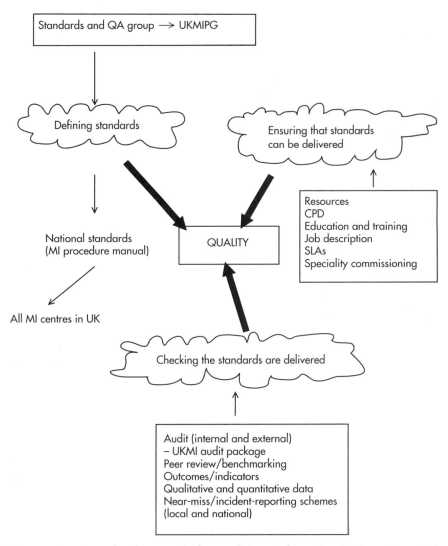

Figure 6.2 A quality framework for medicines information (MI) services. QA, quality assurance; UKMIPG, UK Medicines Information Pharmacists Group; CPD, continuing professional development; SLAs, service level agreements; UKMI, UK Medicines Information.

Risk management has been recognised as an area of crucial importance within the NHS, and within MI services. Many trusts are developing risk management programmes, with which MI services will comply as part of the overall risk management strategy for pharmacy services, and/or through a specific focus on MI services and activities. MI centres in the UK are recommended to develop risk management plans to provide a framework for safe working. The components of such plans are outlined in nationally adopted guidelines [19]. The guidelines identify five risk management standards that are applicable to MI services, the monitoring of which forms the basis for a comprehensive audit process for all MI services. The aim of these standards is to ensure that MI service managers are aware of the potential factors which can contribute to unsafe working practices within MI and that procedures are in place to minimise identified risks. The five standards are listed in Table 6.3.

Table 6.3   Risk management standards for medicines information (MI) services

Standard	*Monitored by*
Standard 1	
1.1 Clear definition of range and availability of services	Availability of appropriate locally agreed policies/documents
1.2 Job descriptions consistent with defined range of services	
1.3 Defined procedure for referral of inappropriate enquiries	
Standard 2	
2.1 Nationally agreed minimum resource levels for books, journals, equipment and staff are met	Part of the enquiry-answering QA programme
Standard 3	
3.1 MI posts have defined 'person specifications'	Availability of appropriate local policies/documents, e.g. IPR and training records
3.2 MI staff have undertaken appropriate training	
3.3 Training needs of MI staff are regularly assessed	
3.4 Competence of MI staff is regularly assessed	
3.5 Delegation of tasks is clearly defined and appropriate	
3.6 Adequate supervision of staff in training is provided	
Standard 4	
4.1 Protocol in use for handling MI enquiries	4.1, 4.2 and 4.4: availability of appropriate policies/documents.
4.2 Guidance on documenting MI enquiries available	
4.3 National enquiry-answering standards met	4.3: as part of enquiry-answering QA audit programme.
4.4 Protocol for production of proactive information in use	
4.5 National standards for MI publications met	4.5: as part of MI publications QA audit programme

(continued)

Reactive

The reactive service is mainly focused on enquiry answering for the broad range of users of the service described previously. Most enquiries to the MI service are directly related to individual patient care, although many are concerned with developing policy and guidelines, pharmacy practice, pharmaceutical issues, pharmaceutical and medicines research and teaching support. The service will answer enquiries on any aspect of the prescribing, supply, formulation and administration of medicines, where possible from an evidence-based perspective. Common types of clinical enquiry are listed in Table 6.4.

Table 6.4 Enquiry types

Enquiry type	Includes
Administration	Route and timing, techniques and equipment
Adverse effects	To all medicines, including over-the-counter (OTC) and alternative therapies, and in all clinical situations (e.g. pregnancy) but excluding poisoning
Alternative therapies	Homeopathic, herbal, aromatherapy and ethnic therapies
Availability	In the UK or abroad for foreign travel
Clinical choice	Best treatment choice, including most appropriate drug in a therapeutic class, for a specified patient or policy
Indications/ contraindications	For what, and in what situations, a drug can be, or should be, used
Dosage	Including in children and in specialist clinical situations, e.g. with renal and hepatic disease
Drug abuse	Often in conjunction with drug abuse specialists
Identification	Ethical, generic, OTC, herbal, homeopathic, veterinary and foreign medicines
Incompatibilities	Normally in intravenous formulations
Interactions	With other drugs, including OTCs, food and laboratory tests
Pharmaceutics	Formulation, excipients, stability and analysis
Pharmacoeconomics	Including cost-effectiveness
Pharmacology/ pharmacokinetics	Mechanism of action and adverse effects and factors associated with metabolism, distribution and excretion
Poisoning/overdose	Normally referred to the Poisons Information Service
Use in specific situations	Pregnancy, breast-feeding, with liver or renal disease, with porphyria, etc.

Providing an effective response to a clinical problem is a multiple-stage process and requires a wide range of skills and knowledge. The main components of the enquiry-answering process can be simplified as:

- contact with the enquirer
- identification of the problem
- acquiring appropriate and adequate background information
- establishing the urgency of the enquiry and prioritising with other enquiries
- retrieval, utilisation and critical appraisal of information relevant to the enquiry. This may include referral to a subject specialist if appropriate
- preparing the response
- presentation of response in most appropriate form, e.g. letter or verbally
- documenting the whole process
- feedback and follow-up if necessary to determine outcome and need for further information.

Guidelines and standard procedures have been established nationally to facilitate this process being undertaken to a consistent and high-quality level across the UK. Enquiry answering is the main activity on which various quality control and audit processes are performed to ensure that the service is meeting its objectives, within a clinical governance framework, in facilitating safe and effective medicines use in patients.

Proactive

The proactive part of the service includes a wide range of outputs, which can be partly or wholly produced by the MI service. The involvement of individual local MI services in these activities varies, dependent on both local need and service resourcing. Proactive outputs aim to provide support to prescribing policy and strategy construction, guideline production and implementation, and education, knowledge and professional development support. The involvement of MI services in these activities includes:

- bulletins and newsletters
- current awareness publications
- horizon scanning for and evidence-based appraisals of new medicines
- clinical guidelines, treatment protocols and patient group directions
- websites (intranet and internet)
- databases of medicines-related data for general use, for example Pharm-line, a bibliographic database on pharmacy practice and therapeutics
- support to primary and secondary care drug and therapeutics committees and formularies

• training and development programmes for MI, therapeutics and critical appraisal skills.

The example of outputs in the area of new drugs serves to illustrate the breadth and penetration of the activities of MI services. Evidence appraisals of new drugs, including new chemical entities, new formulations and new indications, are based on a four-stage national new product scheme. The first two stages are concerned with identifying and tracking new drugs in early clinical development (up to 5 years premarketing) which may have a subsequent impact on prescribing practice in the UK. This activity is also undertaken in collaboration with the NHS National Horizon Scanning Centre. This process supports the third stage, which considers those developments which are later in the development cycle (6–18 months premarketing), for which detailed appraisals of individual technologies and drugs are produced in conjunction with the NHS National Prescribing Centre and distributed throughout the NHS. The fourth stage produces indepth appraisals of key new developments after commercial launch to facilitate the rational use of new medicines and serves as the basis for numerous more local initiatives within individual organisations. This four-stage scheme is shown in more detail in Figure 6.3 and Table 6.5.

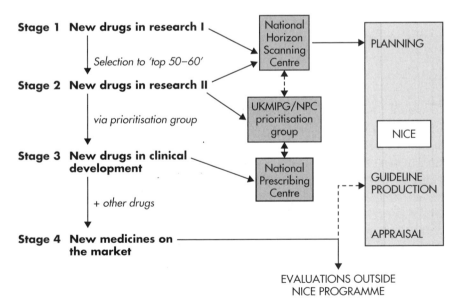

Figure 6.3 New drug entry. UKMIPG, UK Medicines Information Pharmacists Group; NPC, National Prescribing Centre; NICE, National Institute for Clinical Excellence.

Table 6.5 Information on new drugs – summary of stages

Title	Content	Timing	Production/output	Target
Stage 1 New drugs in research (part 1)	Early intelligence on all new drugs likely to reach the UK market that are in late phase II and III trials	Continuous tracking for up to 5 years before marketing	Produced by one regional MI centre with input from others on behalf of UKMIPG	MI pharmacists NHSC
	Information content is brief as many products may never reach the market and early clinical information is scant		Facilitated by direct one-to-one contacts with all major pharmaceutical companies in the UK (through Stage 1 and 2 coordinating centres)	DoH (pharmacy and prescribing branch) Forms the basis of the Stage 2 assessment process
	Contains prediction of possible broad cost implications, where information is available		Output through a 'new products' component of the national MI website, the Stage 1–2 sections being restricted to authorised NHS users only	
	Approximately 500–700 drugs are continuously tracked			

(continued)

Table 6.5 Continued

Title	Content	Timing	Production/output	Target
Stage 2 New drugs in research (part 2)	As Stage 1, but restricted to selected drugs (up to 50–60) which are considered to have greater or closer market potential. These form the basis for the next stages	More limited time scale as intelligence becomes firmer. Probably 6 months to 3 years premarketing	Coordinated by one regional MI centre. Constructed from a priority-rated filter from Stage 1	MI pharmacists D&TCs NHS Horizon Scanning Unit
	Typically drugs are in late phase II, III and preregistration trials	Drugs in this list are continually updated according to the latest intelligence	Contains preliminary information	UKMIPG/NPC collaboration
			Forms the basis of Stage 3 allocations in conjunction with the UKMIPG/NPC prioritisation group	prioritisation group Senior pharmacy managers Prescribing advisers
			Output by quarterly hard-copy listing with regular electronic updating, and as part of the national MI website (see Stage 1)	Directors of public health DoH (pharmacy and prescribing branch)

(continued)

Table 6.5 Continued

Title	Content	Timing	Production/output	Target
Stage 3 New drugs in clinical development	Comprehensive early intelligence evaluations of all new drugs, formulations and indications which are likely to have a significant impact on either prescribing practice or prescribing costs. Minor and 'me-too' drugs are normally omitted	Drugs are identified through Stage 2 and other sources Continuous tracking from about 2 years premarketing, when market potential is able to be assessed	Produced by a group of 10 regional MI centres on behalf of UKMIPG on a rota allocation basis Output as early as information availability permits. May be updated if intelligence changes This stage forms the basis of the NPC/UKMIPG collaboration in which approximately 50% of evaluations have epidemiological and pharmacoeconomic data added by the NPC	Prescribing advisers and other key HA and PCT personnel Senior hospital pharmacy managers MI pharmacists Chief Executives (NHS trusts and health authorities) D&TCs Managers and budget-setters Clinical budget-holders
	Drugs are normally licensed and up to 2 years from marketing			
	Information provides estimates of potential costs, uptake and place in therapeutics, both in primary and secondary care		Also uses drug companies as a source of information	Directors of public health
	Usually excludes specialist drugs, e.g. antineoplastics, vaccines, radiopharmaceuticals, etc		Published jointly with NPC and distributed in hard copy. Web availability under consideration	

(continued)

Table 6.5 Continued

Title	Content	Timing	Production/output	Target
Stage 4 New medicines on the market	Comprehensive, indepth evaluations of most new drugs which are marketed. Currently excludes some drugs in highly specialised clinical areas, e.g. oncology	Drugs identified through Stages 1–3 and through product licence notifications	Currently covers most drugs from Stage 3 and some new, lower-impact drugs	MI pharmacists
				D&TCs
		Allocated for production at time of UK marketing and published within 3 months	New evaluations may be produced for subsequent new indications and presentations	Senior hospital and GP prescribers (when appropriate)
	Includes new chemical entities (including further drugs in existing therapeutic categories), major new formulations and major new indications			Hospital pharmacists
		Also additional drugs which were outside the selection criteria for Stage 3	The impact of, and input into, NICE are taken into account	Prescribing advisers and other key HA and PCT personnel
		Consults drug companies	Published electronically through the national MI website. Hard copy output discontinued December 2000	PCT pharmaceutical advisers and prescribing leads

UKMIPG, UK Medicines Information Pharmacists Group; MI, medicines information; NHS, National Health Service; NPC, National Prescribing Centre; NICE, National Institute for Clinical Excellence; NHSC, National Horizon Scanning Centre; DoH, Department of Health; D&TC, drugs and therapeutics committees; HA, health authority; PCT, primary care trust; GP, general practitioner.

Specialist information services

There are a significant number of subjects which are both specialised by their nature and are frequently referred to due to their nature, which MI pharmacists therefore have to address routinely. Some of these subject areas are of a clinical nature, for example drug use in pregnancy, whilst some are of a pharmaceutical nature, for example medicines which are latex-free. As they are in subject areas which are frequently encountered, a network of MI services providing a specialist information/advisory service in some of these areas has been established over the last 20 years (Table 6.6). This network provides several distinct advantages. Firstly, in clinical areas, it enables the establishment of a depth of understanding and expertise that would not be feasible in every MI service. This includes more comprehensive coverage of the evidence base for that subject, and establishment of clinical 'expert' contacts to augment the information provided. Secondly, for non-clinical subjects, it enables the compilation of comprehensive databases of specialised product information, often with the collaboration of the pharmaceutical industry. In

Table 6.6 Specialised medicines information (MI) services in the UK

Subject		MI service provider
Alternative medicine		Welsh (Cardiff)
Drugs in:	Breast milk and lactation	Trent (Leicester)/West Midlands (Sutton Coldfield)
	Children	Alder Hey Hospital (Liverpool)
	Dentistry	North-west (Liverpool)
	Liver disease	Yorkshire (Leeds)
	Oncology	Royal Marsden Hospital (London)
	Porphyria	Welsh (Cardiff)
	Pregnancy and teratology	Northern and Yorkshire DTC (Newcastle)
	Psychiatry	Maudsley Hospital (London)
	Renal failure	South and West (Bristol)
Drugs of abuse		Wessex (Southampton)
Fridge stability of medicines		North Thames (Northwick Park)
Latex in injections		Nottingham (Queens Medical Centre)
HIV/AIDS		St Mary's/Chelsea and Westminster Hospitals (London)
Toxicology and poisoning		Northern and Yorkshire DTC (Newcastle)/ Northern Ireland (Belfast)

DTC, Drugs and Therapeutic Centre; HIV, human immunodeficiency virus; AIDS, acquired immunodeficiency syndrome.

all cases it provides either a single contact source for users or a single back-up source for MI services, and it reduces a substantial amount of work duplication. The quality of the information is also significantly enhanced. These specialised services were originally based on regional MI centres, but have expanded to encompass the specialities able to be provided from local MI centres based in speciality hospitals or in hospitals providing a high-level speciality in its clinical portfolio. The availability of some of these services is restricted to MI pharmacists only, whilst others have a more open availability and may be wholly or partly web-enabled.

Information resources

MI services require access to a wide range of published information sources to fulfil all the activities outlined. Many activities may require access only to standard reference books or systems that provide relatively static, unchanging information. However, as the role of the MI pharmacist expands, the information sources required are becoming more evidence-based and current, often with use of the primary literature and the main source of information. Whilst textbooks are, and will remain, a valuable source of information, their limitations (cost, currency, completeness) are changing the way in which information and clinical evidence are accessed and utilised. Many standard information sources are now available electronically, commonly on CD-ROM or via the internet, which makes them not only more accessible but increasingly more cost-effective to use.

MI services in the UK have established a minimum information resources standard, i.e. a collection of core information resources which it is considered all MI services must either hold in-house or to which they must have immediate and unrestricted access. Whilst this represents a considerable investment for a local MI service, it forms part of the standard which all such services must meet to be able to provide an acceptable level and quality of service. The resources contained in this minimum standard are continually reviewed and updated for new editions, new titles and obsolescence. The current information resource standard contains reference and textbooks, journals and electronic databases and is common for all MI services. In addition, larger local MI centres, regional MI services and specialist MI services will have a requirement for a wider range of resources which will partly be defined by national standards and partly by service need. One basic premise of information resource use is that only the most recent or current editions of resources should be used. Use of out-of-date resources could lead to the production of unreliable and erroneous information which could result in harm to a patient, or even a legal challenge.

A full, current list of the minimum information resources required can be found at www.ukmi.nhs.uk.

Expanding internet and intranet publishing will increasingly make many of these resources more readily available, often in a form that is 'free to end-user', although this will include current users of MI services. The implications of this shift in the balance of information access and utilisation will have to be taken into account by service providers, including MI services.

In addition to the published resources, MI services will also use in-house collections of commercial and published literature, in-house databases and collections of past outputs (past enquiries, frequently asked questions or FAQs, bulletins, reports and so on) to augment information access.

Information technology

MI services are heavily dependent on all aspects of IT, both to acquire and to disseminate information. The main electronic sources of information are mentioned above. Two key, large bibliographic databases, Medline and Embase, are core resources for accessing the biomedical literature for outputs requiring use of original clinical and pharmaceutical research evidence.

MI services are rapidly moving to the use of electronic distribution of its outputs, both reactive and proactive, through widespread use of e-mail and websites. The IT infrastructure of the NHS is developing slowly but gradually, enabling all main users of MI services to receive and access MI electronically. This is rapidly becoming the standard method of distributing tailored information to specific users. Also, MI services are increasingly putting the proactive outputs of the service on websites, either intranet and/or internet, for both immediate and subsequent archived access by users.

The main focus of web-based development is a national MI website, www.ukmi.nhs.uk, which aims to provide a one-stop resource for MI in the UK. This website provides a wide range of information, including clinical MI, current awareness, training and research resources and a single source of all strategic and operational policies and MI guidelines. It also gives access to all the major outputs of regional MI centres, through a direct portal to websites of regional MI services. The national MI website is augmented with a UK-wide e-mail discussion group, MI-UK, which serves as a means of MI pharmacists communicating and sharing experiences and problems.

Staffing and training

As with most areas of professional practice, the most important resource of MI services is its staff. As previously described, MI services are normally managed by experienced clinical pharmacists with specialist training to develop the additional skills and knowledge required. Training in MI skills and techniques is started formally at the preregistration stage, with most pharmacy graduates undergoing specific MI training before registration, which also meets the requirements of the Royal Pharmaceutical Society for pharmacists' competencies. After registration this is normally augmented with further training, both formally and through placements in local or regional MI centres. Developing clinical and problem-solving skills provides an ongoing development of MI-related skills, which can be applied at a ward/patient level through the provision of clinical pharmacy and then through a more formal MI service setting.

Pharmacists working more formally in an MI service, with a specific responsibility for providing support to clinical pharmacy and associated MI activities, are then normally exposed to more formal MI training on a national basis. In the UK, a structured training programme is in place, starting with a National Introductory MI Training Course which introduces the pharmacist to the range of skills and activities relevant to an MI specialist. Entry to this course requires a basic level of predetermined competencies acquired through structured work experience. This level of training aims to enable the trainee to:

- understand and apply the skills, knowledge and resources to provide clinically oriented MI
- apply the basic principles of searching electronic sources of information, in particular Medline and the internet
- know the strengths and weaknesses of the key MI databases, including the internet
- apply basic statistical tests to clinical trial data
- identify the key components of clinical trial design and apply these to critical appraisal of the literature
- know the necessary verbal communication skills required to deliver an effective MI service
- identify legal and ethical problems that may be encountered when providing MI

- know the principles of clinical governance, and in particular risk management and quality, and apply these to the provision of MI.

This training is supported by the availability of a national training and procedure manual for MI services [15]. More advanced training to develop skills, knowledge and effective use of resources is then provided to suit the needs of the individual and the service.

The whole training strategy is supported by a national competency framework for MI, introduced in 2001, the aim of which is to 'identify the competencies that individuals working in MI either have, or need to develop, in order to perform their work effectively now and in the future' [20]. The framework is used to:

- facilitate continuing professional development at an individual level
- help managers and MI pharmacists identify ongoing training and development needs
- provide a framework to support local recruitment and appraisal processes.

Although pharmacists have been the principal component of the human resource of MI services in the past, other professional groups are now being considered, and actively deployed, in MI services to support and provide some of its activities. In particular, experienced pharmacy technicians are now considered to be appropriate staff to utilise in the service, as they are in many other areas of clinical pharmacy practice. Appropriate technicians, once identified, are trained through a rigorously controlled programme which includes core training, in-house work, supervised work, experience, development of a personal work portfolio, continuous assessment, a probationary period and subsequent accreditation as an MI technician. Accredited technicians can then assume some responsibilities within the enquiry-answering process. Seven common enquiry types are considered appropriate, for which MI technicians can have a substantive responsibility, although the final responsibility for the overall process remains with the MI pharmacist. These are:

- tablet and capsule identification
- availability of medicines
- formulation and stability (excluding parenteral)
- interactions
- adverse effects/Committee on Safety of Medicines data
- complementary medicines
- travel medicine.

Routine activity within these seven designated subject areas is covered by the accreditation process. However, MI technicians can be involved in other enquiry types and other MI activities as long as adequate training has been undertaken and risk management issues assessed.

The future

Development of MI technicians' activities and responsibilities will be an important feature of future service development which will take account of skill mix, recruitment and clinical competence issues. Other professional groups, including information scientists, life science graduates, librarians and others, may also have roles to fulfil in future MI services which are yet to be defined.

Conclusion

The activities and skills described in this chapter illustrate the broad and crucial role played both in pharmacy and in the broader NHS by MI services. The MI service has developed as a respected and valued support service to health professions, in all health care sectors. It has roles as diverse as supporting and maximising the effectiveness of individual patient care to facilitating the development of national medicines-related policy. MI services in the UK are frequently cited as a role model for health care systems outside the UK, but the unique nature of the NHS has been the main factor in the way in which MI services have developed as a self-supporting network with operational and strategic roles at local and national levels.

Advances in IT are changing the way in which MI services both gather and disseminate information. The advent of electronic prescribing in hospitals will further add to the changes that MI services will have to encompass and support. No matter how powerful and extensive IT-driven health information becomes, these developments will only be additional tools to the MI practitioner – tools to increase the efficiency and effectiveness of service delivery and enhance user accessibility. MI practitioners, pharmacists and technicians will still be the ultimate source of quality, critically assessed and tailored information on medicines. To achieve this, however, the service will have to remain constantly vigilant to developments in the NHS which change its user base and the opportunities for new 'customers', to developments in IT through which to deliver its service, to new players in the health care information market with which it will develop collaborative and partnership arrangements, and to new developments in therapeutics and medicines-related health care technologies which will constantly change its knowledge requirements. Underpinning all this will be the users of the service, from bedside to board room, who are treating patients and devising health care policy.

References

1. Hall N, chair. *Report of the Working Party Investigating the Hospital Pharmaceutical Service.* London: HMSO, 1970.
2. Anonymous. Leeds hospital plans full time pharmacy service. *Pharm J* 1971; 207: 561.
3. Rogers M L, Barrett C W. The drug information centre at the London Hospital. *Pharm J* 1972; 209: 37–39.
4. Anonymous. Report of the working party on drug information services. *Pharm J* 1974; 213: 297–301.
5. Leach F N. The regional drug information service: a factor in health care? *BMJ* 1978; 178: 766–768.
6. Anonymous. Getting the information we need – how drug information centres can help. *Drug Ther Bull* 1978; 16: 41–43.
7. Smith J C, McNulty H. The national drug information network. *Pharm J* 1982; 228: 67–69.
8. Proudlove C R, Smith J D C, Breckenridge A M. Medical awareness and usage of a regional drug information service. *Pharm J* 1983; 230: 394–396.
9. Hands D, Judd A, Golightly P W *et al.* Drug information and advisory services – past, present and future. *Pharm J* 1999; 262: 160–162.
10. Jenkins P. Secretary of State views the pharmaceutical scene and outlines his policy. *Pharm J* 1979; 223: 240.
11. Audit Commission. *A Prescription for Improvement – Towards more Rational Prescribing in General Practice.* London: Audit Commission/HMSO, 1994.
12. Department of Health. *Memorandum of Understanding on Appraisal of Health Interventions.* London: Department of Health, 1999.
13. UKMIPG. *Better Information for Managing Medicines – A Strategy for Pharmacy's Medicines Information in the NHS.* UK Medicines Information Pharmacists Group, 2000.
14. Royal Pharmaceutical Society of Great Britain. *Medicines, Ethics and Practice – A Guide for Pharmacists,* 26th edn. London: RPSGB, 2002.
15. UKDIPG. Legal and ethical aspects of drug information. In: Judd A, ed. *UK Drug Information Manual,* 4th edn. UKDIPG, 1997: 3.1–3.16.
16. Department of Health. *A First Class Service: Quality in the New NHS.* London: The Stationery Office, 1998.
17. Royal Pharmaceutical Society of Great Britain. *Achieving Excellence in Pharmacy Through Clinical Governance.* London: RPSGB, 1999.
18. Strategy and Quality Assurance Working Party UKMIPG. *Clinical Governance: A Briefing Paper for Medicines Information Services.* 2000.
19. UKDIPG. Risk management in drug information. In: Judd A, ed. *UK Drug Information Manual,* 4th edn. UKDIPG, 1997: 16.1–16.25.

20.   Picton C. *A Competency Framework in Medicines Information*. UKMIPG, 2001.

Further reading

Better Information for Managing Medicines – A Strategy for Pharmacy's Medicines Information in the NHS. UK Medicines Information Pharmacists Group, 2000.

Hands D, Judd A, Golightly P W *et al.* Drug information and advisory services – past, present and future. *Pharm J* 1999; 262: 160–162.

7

Clinical pharmacy services

Damian Child and Jonathan Cooke

The ability of any health care organisation to optimise the use of medicines is called medicines management.

Definition of medicines management

Medicines management in hospitals encompasses the entire way that medicines are selected, procured, delivered, prescribed, administered and reviewed to optimise the contribution that medicines make to producing informed and desired outcomes of patient care [1].

Ward pharmacy

One of the differences between hospital and community pharmacy is the location of the patient and how this affects the dynamics of providing pharmaceutical care. Most hospitals provide their pharmaceutical services to patients on (but not exclusively) wards of various kinds. Thus in order to deliver care the pharmacist needs to visit the ward and interact with the patient, doctor, nurse and others, as well as have access to consult and contribute to the patient's medical records.

Pharmaceutical presence on wards allows dialogue with patients and professionals in addition to ensuring supplies of medicines are adequate for the patients' needs, and that medicines are stored appropriately and safely. Pharmacy technicians, assistants and others work with ward staff to provide effective supply of commonly used items and, with the pharmacists, are increasingly leading the introduction of the reuse of patients' own drugs (PODs) schemes and, where appropriate, patient self-medication.

The importance of communicating requests for medicines and the need to record administration of medicines have led to the universal usage of the ward prescription chart. Various reports on the value of recording the prescription and administration of medicines emanated from situations where there was no record of them having been given. Requiring nurses and doctors to record the administration of medicines offered the rudiments of an audit trail for medicines.

The design and use of these charts have consumed much time and energy from a variety of clinicians in order to produce a hybrid document that serves the multiple purposes of conveying:

- patient details such as identification, age, weight, gender, allergies
- prescribing details such as medicine, form, dose, route and frequency of administration and previous medicines
- medicine administration details including who administered (nurse, doctor, patient), when and by which route. It also serves to indicate when a medicine has **not** been given.

Figure 7.1 is an extract from a typical inpatient medicines chart. These important sets of data are essential for the efficient and effective delivery of pharmaceutical care to the patient. They will form the basis for the development of electronic prescribing systems within the National Health Service (NHS), as outlined in *Information for Health* [2].

History

Until the mid-1960s, hospital pharmacists were mostly engaged in traditional pharmaceutical activities such as dispensing and manufacturing [3]. However, the increasing range and sophistication of medicines available, awareness of medication errors and the widespread use of ward-based prescription charts brought pharmacists out of the dispensary and on to the wards in increasing numbers.

This was initially described as 'ward pharmacy', and was mostly a retrospective process with the emphasis on the safe and timely supply of medicines in response to medical and nursing demands. However, the service quickly evolved into something significantly more proactive, seeing pharmacists interacting with patients and other health care professionals and directly intervening in the patient care process [4]. The growth in these services over the 1970s and 1980s was said to represent a change in hospital pharmacy from product orientation to patient orientation and was formally acknowledged as 'clinical pharmacy' in the 1986 Nuffield Report [3]. The report welcomed these changes and recommended an increased role for hospital pharmacists through the development of clinical pharmacy services.

HMR 111(E)1   Sheet No.

PRESCRIPTION SHEET

OR USE ADDRESS-O-GRAPH PLATE

Hospital   Ward

ALLERGIES, DRUG SENSITIVITIES AND RELEVANT THERAPY

UNIT No.

SURNAME (Block letters)

FIRST NAMES

DATE OF BIRTH

FIX CONTINUATION (HMR 111J) HERE

DATE	ONCE ONLY & PREMEDICANT DRUGS	Dose	Route	Time	Signature	Given at & Initials	Pharm.

AS REQUIRED PRESCRIPTIONS (including post-operative drugs)

Administration Record   FIX CONTINUATION (HMR 111F) HERE

Date	Time	Dose	Given	Date	Time	Dose	Given	Date	Time	Dose	Given

DRUG

Route	Dose	Date	MAXIMUM NUMBER OF DOSES OF CONTROLLED DRUG

Signature   Pharmacist

SPECIAL INSTRUCTIONS

DRUG

Route	Dose	Date	MAXIMUM NUMBER OF DOSES OF CONTROLLED DRUG

Signature   Pharmacist

SPECIAL INSTRUCTIONS

DRUG

Route	Dose	Date	MAXIMUM NUMBER OF DOSES OF CONTROLLED DRUG

Signature   Pharmacist

SPECIAL INSTRUCTIONS

DRUG

Route	Dose	Date	MAXIMUM NUMBER OF DOSES OF CONTROLLED DRUG

Signature   Pharmacist

SPECIAL INSTRUCTIONS

DRUG

Route	Dose	Date	MAXIMUM NUMBER OF DOSES OF CONTROLLED DRUG

Signature   Pharmacist

SPECIAL INSTRUCTIONS

Please read instructions on Page One

Figure 7.1 Prescription sheet.

Clinical pharmacy

The recommendations made in the Nuffield Report were officially recognised in a 1988 Health Services circular, *The Way Forward for Hospital Pharmaceutical Services* [5]. This document outlined the main aims of the Department of Health with respect to hospital pharmacy:

> The achievement of better patient care and financial savings through the more cost effective use of medicines and improved use of pharmaceutical services obtained by implementing a clinical pharmacy service.

A number of key areas where pharmacist input could assist other clinicians and benefit patients were highlighted, including contribution to prescribing decisions, monitoring and modifying drug therapy, counselling patients and involvement in clinical trials. The document acknowledged that by helping to ensure patient safety and appropriate use of medicines, clinical pharmacy services could prove to be cost-effective.

As clinical pharmacy services expanded, there was increasing specialisation, with the expertise of individual pharmacists in certain therapeutic areas contributing to more significant developments in service provision. The speed of progress was demonstrated in a review undertaken in the early 1990s, which showed that the majority of NHS hospitals in the UK provided clinical pharmacy services and most hospital pharmacists participated in ward-based clinical pharmacy activities [4]. However, the range of clinical pharmacy services varied enormously, from almost 100% of hospitals having pharmacists who monitored drug therapy, to less than 10% for services such as infection control, clinical audit or medical staff education [6]. Since then, the widespread development of clinical pharmacy services has continued, with significant expansion in the number and range of services provided at most hospitals.

Wide variations in the extent and nature of hospital clinical pharmacy services were also noted in the Nuffield Report and large differences still exist across much of the UK [1, 7]. This lack of uniformity does not just apply to clinical pharmacy, but covers almost every aspect of hospital pharmacy services. The absence of specific directions from the Department of Health and from the pharmacy profession, coupled with the varying degrees of success with which individual pharmacy managers in each hospital have been able to develop services, has allowed diversity to flourish. The most recent survey of hospital pharmacy services still showed wide variations in the proportion of time spent on clinical pharmacy activities, ranging from less than 30% of pharmacist time at some hospitals to over 70% of pharmacist time at others [1]. The report recommended that hospitals undertake reviews of their staffing levels and consider whether there were adequate resources to provide all aspects of clinical pharmacy services, so it is likely that the national figures on implementation of clinical pharmacy services will be changing for some time.

Pharmaceutical care

In 1990, the introduction of the concept of pharmaceutical care by American pharmacists Hepler and Strand led to further developments in clinical pharmacy services [8]. This was defined as 'the responsible provision of drug therapy for the purpose of achieving definite outcomes which improve the patient's quality of life'. The definition included pharmacist input in the design, implementation and monitoring of a therapeutic plan, in collaboration with the patient and other health care professionals, and helped to change the focus of clinical pharmacy activities from processes to therapeutic outcomes. However, despite widespread acceptance, use of the term 'pharmaceutical care' in the UK does not always follow the rigorous definition of Hepler and Strand but is often used simply to imply a patient-focused approach to clinical pharmacy practice [7].

Pharmacy, by definition, is a clinical profession and the term 'clinical pharmacy' is somewhat outdated as the NHS now recognises that the term 'clinician' refers to all health care staff involved with the care of patients. A definition of clinician from *A First Class Service, Quality in the New NHS* [9] is:

> those directly involved in the care and treatment of patients, including doctors, dentists, nurses, midwives, health visitors, pharmacists, opticians, chiropodists, radiographers, orthoptists, physiotherapists, dietitians, occupational therapists, medical laboratory scientific officers, orthotists and prosthetists, therapists, speech and language therapists and all other health professionals.

Thus pharmacy is a patient-centred service where the pharmacist is a key member of the clinical team. Pharmacists should be involved with all aspects of the 'patient journey' though the hospital (Table 7.1).

Table 7.1 Clinical pharmacy and the patient journey: roles for the clinical pharmacist

Before admission

Preadmission clinics – reviewing previous medications, assessing allergies, explaining medicines that will be used in addition

Contribution to integrated-care pathways (ICPs) – writing guidelines and contributing to formulary monographs

Liaison with community pharmacists, general practitioners and community nurses Involvement with patient groups – teaching about the importance of medicines

Education of patients, the general public and children about the importance of medicines

On admission

Medical admission unit – taking medication histories, reviewing patients' medicines and obtaining consent for patients' own drugs

General and specialist wards – as above

During stay

Promoting the formulary management system

Contributing to selection of medicines, formulation, dose

Monitoring response to treatment

Modifying doses in response to blood levels or changes in renal and liver function and in consideration of extremes of age

Looking for unwanted effects and interactions of medicines

Reporting adverse drug reactions to medicines

Contributing to local incident-reporting systems

Liaising with other clinicians on the wards

Education and training programmes

Auditing use of medicines

Undertaking research on the use of medicines

On discharge

Advising and informing patients on their medication

Writing discharge prescriptions

Liaising with primary care teams

Activities that are components of the delivery of pharmaceutical care in hospitals

Prescription monitoring

The core of pharmacists' contribution to appropriate prescribing and medication use is made whilst undertaking near-patient clinical pharmacy activities. Checking and monitoring patients' prescriptions on hospital wards is frequently the starting point for this process and on most hospital wards the prescription card and clinical observation charts (temperature, pulse rate, blood pressure, etc.) are kept at the end of the patients' beds. This allows the clinical pharmacist to interact with the patient whilst reviewing the contents of the prescription.

The prescription is reviewed for medication dosing errors, appropriateness of administration route, drug interactions, prescription ambiguities, inappropriate prescribing and many other potential problems. Formal assessments of prescription charts in hospitals have shown that there are wide variations in the quality of prescribing and pharmacists have been able to identify and resolve many clinical problems [10–12].

Patients can be questioned on their medication histories, including allergies and intolerances, efficacy of prescribed treatment, side-effects and adverse drug reactions (ADRs). The routine presence of medical and nursing staff on the ward allows the pharmacist to communicate easily with other members of the health care team who value the prescription monitoring service that clinical pharmacists provide [13, 14]. The patients' notes are also accessible, to enable the pharmacist both to check important information that may affect their health care and to record details of any clinical pharmacy input made.

Prescribing advice to medical and nursing staff

Prescribing advice can be provided by medicines information pharmacists within the pharmacy department or by pharmacists undertaking their clinical pharmacy duties in patient areas such as the wards or outpatient clinics. This latter role may also include attendance at medical ward rounds [15]. The advice given can include help with choice of medicine, dose, method of administration, side-effects, interactions, monitoring requirements and many other aspects of medicines use. Studies examining prescribing advice given by clinical pharmacists have shown high rates of acceptance from medical staff, demonstrating that the role is both valued and effective [16, 17].

Medication errors and adverse drug reaction reporting

Despite the important role of clinical pharmacy services, patients receiving drug therapy may still experience unintended harm or injury as a result of medication errors or from ADRs. Adverse events (from any cause) occur in around 10% of all hospital admissions and medication errors account for one-quarter of all the incidents which threaten patient safety [18]. It is also acknowledged that hospitals have recognised and documented only a small proportion of these adverse events [18]. Important lessons can be learned from analysis of medication-related incidents and from 'near-misses' (i.e. those that do not develop sufficiently to result in patient harm or are detected prior to patient harm). Chapter 9 will consider these issues in further detail.

Contributing to the avoidance or resolution of adverse medication events is an important part of any hospital pharmacist's clinical duties. This requires a multisystem approach often incorporated into a hospital's clinical risk management strategy. Even when the prescribed and administered treatment is correct and no errors have occurred, a small proportion of patients can still suffer from ADRs. Clinical pharmacists have an important role to play in the detection and management of ADRs and, more recently, directly reporting ADRs to the Committee on Safety of Medicines via the 'Yellow Card' scheme. Their involvement can help to increase the number of ADR reports made, particularly those involving serious reaction [19, 20]. However, even in hospitals with formal ADR schemes, gross underreporting of reactions still remains a major problem [21].

Medication history taking

An increasingly important role for clinical pharmacists is medication history taking for patients on admission to hospital. Many problems on admission stem from incomplete or inaccurate information on the medicines that patients are taking. Published work suggests that pharmacists are able to take more accurate medication histories than medical staff [22, 23].

The pharmacist collates and records information on all medications the patient is taking, including non-prescription medicines (over-the-counter products or herbal remedies), in addition to those that have been prescribed by a doctor. The pharmacist can also question the patient on concordance with prescribed treatment, check patients' own medicines to ensure suitability for reuse in hospital PODs and self-medication schemes and help to identify whether or not an admission is due to prescribing errors or ADRs. Pharmacy technicians are increasingly involved in supporting these roles and in contributing to medication checking and POD schemes. Their roles are discussed further below; chapter 3 discusses supply systems, including POD schemes.

For planned admissions to hospital (for example, for routine surgery), the medication history-taking role can be moved to an earlier stage in the patient care process. Preadmission clinics have traditionally been used to assess patients' suitability for surgery, but are also increasingly used to make other preparations for admission. Clinical pharmacists can work alongside medical and nursing staff, to help ensure that full and accurate details of medication are recorded and that patients either bring their own medication with them on admission or medicines not routinely stocked by the hospital pharmacy can be ordered in advance [23, 24].

Patient education and counselling, including achieving concordance

One of the key themes of the NHS plan is empowering patients to take an active role in managing their own care [25]. Helping patients to understand their medicines and how to take them is a major feature of clinical pharmacy. Patient compliance, defined as adherence to the regimen of treatment recommended by the doctor, has been a concern of health care professionals for some time [26]. Adherence to treatment, particularly for long-term chronic conditions, can be poor and tends to worsen as the number of medicines and complexity of treatment regimens increase.

More recently, use of the term 'compliance' in the context of medication has been criticised because it implied that patients must simply follow the doctor's orders, rather than making properly informed decisions about their health care. The term 'concordance' has been proposed as a more appropriate description of the situation:

> Concordance is a new approach to the prescribing and taking of medicines. It is an agreement reached after negotiation between a patient and health care professional that respects the beliefs and wishes of the patient in determining whether, when and how medicines are taken [27].

This change in approach aims to optimise the benefits of treatment by helping patients and clinicians collaborate in a therapeutic partnership. However, if patients are to make informed choices, then the need for comprehensive patient education becomes more pressing.

Many surveys have found that patients often know little about the medicines they are taking. Several studies examining patient counselling and education have shown that clinical pharmacists can help to improve patients' knowledge of their treatment [28, 29]. The contribution made can also improve patient adherence to treatment [28, 30]. Improved adherence should lead to improved outcomes and evidence has been collected to demonstrate this [28, 30, 31].

In addition to providing face-to-face education and counselling on medicines, clinical pharmacists can also help patients by contributing to the preparation of written material, audiovisual demonstrations or with the aid of computer programs [32–35].

Concordance

How patients take their medicines is a crucial component of whether they will respond. Key to this is the health beliefs of the individual and the partnerships with their health care providers that are necessary in order to ensure this happens.

Society is moving away from a paternalistic approach to health care to a more empowered one. Thus, when a patient used to accept a course of treatment obediently it is now negotiated and options, risks and benefits are discussed and, where necessary, consent is obtained. Thus there is a greater need for information and education of the patient and/or carer in order for them to be able to make informed decisions about their treatment.

Concordance with treatment is dependent on a complex interplay of beliefs, trust and understanding, some of which can be influenced by a pharmacist. For example:

1. Individual patients must appreciate that they have a problem.
2. They have to accept the accuracy of the diagnosis.
3. They have to agree common goals for the agreed treatment with the health care provider.
4. They have to understand how to take the medicine, how to tell whether it is working and what to do if unwanted events occur (side-effects and adverse effects).
5. They need to know what to do when their supply runs out.
6. They have to remember to take the medicine.

Points 1 and 2 are effectively the responsibility of the doctor or **independent prescriber** and would not require the input of a pharmacist unless they could identify a medicine-related reason in the diagnostic process, as may sometimes be the case in liver and skin diseases.

Point 3 can be influenced by the pharmacist, e.g. medicines, versus another intervention, e.g. surgery or choice between different medicines. This might be affected by coexisting disease states, for example, diabetes, angina, asthma. Guidelines set within a formulary might assist this process.

Points 4–6 are the responsibility of the pharmacist who will need to implement information and education programmes to support the patient. These might include group sessions, patient information leaflets, supplementary labels and patient self-administration whilst in hospital. A common source of information is the internet and this has many useful sites. However there are other sites where quality is dubious and others where information is dangerous.

Patient empowerment is becoming a focus for both governments and the pharmaceutical industry. Thus in the UK, as in many countries, there is a gradual process of deregulating medicines from prescription-only to pharmacy (over-the-counter) and total general availability. Direct-to-consumer advertising (DCA) of prescription medicines is now prevalent in North America and exceeds the budgets spent on advertising to professionals [36].

Self-administration schemes

Schemes which allow patients to self-administer their medicines whilst in hospital have been attempted in selected groups or settings [37, 38]. The purpose of the schemes is to ensure that patients can deal with their medicines prior to discharge; the schemes could also reduce the dependence of patients on nurses whilst on the wards. Considerable effort may be required to assess patients' suitability and the clinical pharmacist can support nursing staff in this process. A POD scheme, though not essential, can be a useful precursor to such schemes.

Pharmacokinetics and therapeutic drug level monitoring

Pharmacokinetics addresses the absorption, distribution, metabolism and excretion of drugs in patients. A sound knowledge of the pharmacokinetic profiles of different drugs enables the pharmacist to assess the dosing requirements for certain drugs in patients in extremes of age and in the presence of impairment of kidney and liver function. Clinically important drug interactions and adverse reactions can sometimes be predicted. Dosing calculations of aminoglycoside antibiotics are usually made by employing pharmacokinetic principles.

A number of medicines in common use have a narrow therapeutic index. That is, the difference between the lowest effective dose and a potentially toxic dose can be quite small. In many cases it is necessary or desirable to undertake therapeutic drug level monitoring (TDM) to ensure that patients can be treated safely. TDM services include the measurement of drug levels in the patient's blood and the application of clinical pharmacokinetics to optimise drug therapy. There is a wide range of medicines that fall into this category, but TDM services typically include aminoglycoside antibiotics, anticonvulsants, ciclosporin, digoxin, lithium and theophylline. Monitoring drug levels in patients can also provide an important indicator as to whether they are taking their medicine.

Clinical pharmacy input into TDM services can range from the provision of simple advice to other clinicians on when to take samples and how to interpret results, to fully fledged services that may also include collection and laboratory analysis of the blood sample [39–41].

Education and training others

As hospital clinical pharmacy services expanded, there was a growing recognition of the need for postgraduate training for pharmacists. A full-time MSc course in Clinical Pharmacy started at Manchester University in 1978 and others quickly followed [42, 43]. This included the development of part-time courses, which resulted in a significant increase in the numbers of pharmacists being able to receive postgraduate training in clinical pharmacy. The majority of UK NHS hospitals now employ clinical pharmacists with advanced postgraduate qualifications. The training and education that hospital pharmacists receive are covered in more detail in chapter 13. Clinical pharmacy services also include the regular provision of training and education for other health care staff at most hospitals – a service that is valued highly [4].

Medicines formularies

The role of the pharmacist in the development of medicines formularies is covered in more detail in chapter 8. Pharmacists providing clinical services are responsible for ensuring that doctors' prescribing practices comply with formulary recommendations. Clinical pharmacists' detailed knowledge of medicines and the regular contact they have with doctors, nurses and patients mean that they are ideally placed to influence prescribing on the wards. A key feature of successful medicines rationalisation is the ongoing communication between prescribers and pharmacists who encourage self-audit and peer review [44].

Professional and clinical audit

The range and complexity of health care services being provided to patients mean that there is now a need to look more critically at the effectiveness of what is being delivered [45]. Professional self-examination in health care dates back more than a century, but the widespread implementation of clinical audit started in earnest in the early 1990s [46]. This resulted from a number of important factors:

- public expectations that professionals can deliver and maintain high standards of care
- government pressures to make health care professionals more accountable
- the need to enhance and maintain professional credibility.

Clinical pharmacists can be involved in many different types of audit. These may range from topics including audit of clinical services themselves (for example, clinical pharmacy interventions) or may examine which treatments are used and how they are implemented within the framework of drug use evaluations. Audit aims to improve patient outcomes by examining how current clinical practice compares to agreed standards of care, implementing any changes necessary and then re-examining practice to ensure that real improvements have been made.

The most obvious benefits of good clinical audit include improvements in the quality of service and treatment. In addition, enhanced professional standing, improved communication with colleagues, increased knowledge, improved work satisfaction, publication opportunities and even promotion have all been put forward as other positive aspects that should encourage health care staff to get involved.

> Clinical audit is pivotal in patient care: it brings together professionals from all sectors of health care to consider clinical evidence, promote education and research, develop and implement clinical guidelines, enhance information management skills and contribute to better management of resources – all with the aim of improving the quality of care of patients [47].

Anticoagulant services

Clinical pharmacy input into anticoagulant therapy is now a widely accepted part of clinical practice in many hospitals. Some anticoagulant services were initially set up as collaborative ventures with medical staff, but many services are now managed by pharmacists [48]. Although the exact nature of services provided by the pharmacist may vary slightly from hospital to hospital, the role of the pharmacist in anticoagulation has been clearly established:

- ensuring complete documentation and referral information is present
- interviewing patients and assessing factors which may affect anticoagulant control, particularly disease states and drug interactions

- monitoring and adjusting anticoagulant doses to maintain international normalised ratio (INR) within the agreed therapeutic targets
- identifying clinical problems requiring referral to a physician
- patient counselling and education
- providing a regular point of contact for patients with concerns about their treatment
- day-to-day clinic management
- training and education for physicians and pharmacists
- research and audit.

Clinical pharmacists can provide high-quality cost-effective anticoagulant services for both hospital inpatients and outpatients. Evaluations of services provided show that pharmacist anticoagulant control is at least as good as, and in some cases better than, that achieved by medical staff [48, 49].

Outpatient clinical pharmacy services

The traditional role of outpatient prescription dispensing is being replaced in many hospitals by clinical pharmacy input into the clinics themselves. This practice follows the logic that hospitals should only dispense medicines to those outpatients in immediate need. This allows hospitals to utilise some of the resources saved to implement more beneficial pharmacy services such as confirming medication history details, patient counselling and education and providing prescribing advice to medical staff.

In many hospitals pharmacists now actively manage medication for selected outpatients, including those on anticoagulation (see above), lithium, rheumatology medication, lipid-lowering agents and many others [50–52].

Primary/secondary care interface

Outreach pharmacy services such as those supplied to health centres and clinics are covered in chapter 10. However, good-quality clinical pharmacy services do not begin and end at the traditional barriers between hospital and community practice. The overall aim of such services is to provide patients with a smooth transition as they move between the primary and secondary care sectors during admission to or discharge from hospital, a process often described as 'seamless care'. Firstly, the efficient and accurate transfer of information is an essential part of this process if unintended changes in medication are to be avoided. This involves good communication links between other hospital colleagues, general practitioners and community pharmacists in addition to direct patient contact.

Other clinical pharmacy services that can contribute to seamless care include patient follow-up and domiciliary visiting, coordinating appropriate use of compliance aids, the availability of telephone helplines for patients and the establishment of joint primary/secondary care treatment protocols [53].

Pain management

In the past, clinical decisions regarding patients' pain management were normally left to medical staff, but in recent years there have been significant increases in the use of multidisciplinary clinical teams to manage pain, with widespread collaboration between medical, nursing, pharmacy and other staff.

Clinical pharmacy input to pain management typically falls into the categories of acute pain management, commonly in postoperative patients and/or in association with the use of patient-controlled analgesia (PCA) devices, and chronic pain management, most notably in the field of palliative care [54–56].

Clinical pharmacy input to a hospital's pain team can include making recommendations on drug choice, establishing drug therapy protocols, enhancing patient understanding and compliance through education and counselling, monitoring patient outcomes, helping to achieve better pain and symptom control and education of other health care staff. In addition, pharmacists involved in PCA services can help to select the infusion devices to be used, program dosing details into the devices and set them up to deliver effective analgesia to patients.

Increasing role of the pharmacy technician in clinical pharmacy services

The role of pharmacy technicians is already well established in departmental activities such as dispensing and aseptic services. However, the expansion of clinical pharmacy services in hospital would not be possible without the additional support that can be provided by hospital pharmacy technicians.

In a similar manner to the way in which ward pharmacy services provided by pharmacists evolved into clinical pharmacy, pharmacy technicians' roles are becoming increasingly clinical in nature and can include a wide range of activities [57–59]. Some activities are:

- inpatient counselling
- checking medication in POD schemes
- medicines information
- involvement in clinical trials
- preparation of medicines formularies and guidelines
- training and education
- liaison with clinical teams on medicines management and expenditure.

Services linked to clinical specialities

In much the same way that clinical specialities are firmly established in medicine and surgery, the same is now true for clinical pharmacy. This has been helped by the manner in which clinical specialities have been managed in hospitals, often divided into divisions or directorates along clinical lines, to which a pharmacist can be attached. Part of the responsibilities for such pharmacists will be managerial and financial, supporting the management of the medicines budget and contributing to the preparation of business cases for new drugs. There are also well-recognised clinical roles and a selection are described below, although this list is far from exhaustive.

General medicine (including care of the elderly)

Many of the activities undertaken by clinical pharmacists in general medicine are shared with a wide range of other clinical specialities. Numerous factors can influence both the choice of treatment given and the patient's response to that treatment, so ensuring that all patients' pharmaceutical care needs are met is often a difficult task. Medical patients requiring admission to hospital rarely have just one condition or disease state, particularly as patients get older. The expert advice that can be provided by clinical pharmacists becomes increasingly important as the drug treatment becomes ever more complex. Even within the discipline of medicine there is often increasing subspecialisation in clinical pharmacy, mirroring that found in medical practice.

Typical services provided to general medical patients can include the following:

- Comprehensive medication history taking. This is particularly important, as at the time of many emergency medical admissions, patients may not have brought in their medicines or an accurate list, previous hospital notes may not yet be available and the general practitioner surgery may be closed. The clinical pharmacist can confirm these details once the patient has been admitted, to ensure that the baseline prescription on admission is accurate.

- Daily prescription review to identify and resolve prescribing errors, side-effects and ADRs. These are common yet frequently underrecognised problems in patients prescribed multiple drug treatments.
- Advice to other health care colleagues on safe and appropriate prescribing, administration and monitoring of medicines.
- Organisation of medication supply. Although not strictly a clinical activity, this is frequently undertaken by clinical pharmacists in conjunction with their other ward-based duties. However, pharmacy technicians are increasingly taking on this role and the introduction of electronic prescribing and automated dispensing systems is also likely to remove this from the list of pharmacist responsibilities.
- Review and rationalisation of treatment regimens, including advice on cessation of medicines no longer required.
- Patient counselling and education, including the provision of patient aids where appropriate, as well as medication charts and monitored-dose systems to aid compliance.
- Discharge planning for patients, including communication with primary care colleagues where appropriate.
- Speciality-wide medicines management activities, including identification and introduction of new drug treatment options, formulary and guidelines preparation and implementation, financial planning and many other activities.
- Education and training of other health care professionals.

The National Service Framework for older people has a substantial section on medicines-related issues. Although these have important implications for primary care staff, the clinical pharmacist in secondary care also has a role to play [60]. Clinical pharmacy input to the overall care of general medical patients of all ages results in many benefits to both patients and to the hospital service as a whole. These can include reducing medication errors, improving patient concordance with treatment, speeding discharge from hospital and reducing medication costs [61–63].

Surgery

Although surgeons may have expert knowledge of the medicines that they use most frequently, in common with colleagues in most other specialities there are many clinical areas in which they welcome the assistance of clinical pharmacists.

Whether or not patients' long-term drug treatment should be continued during the perioperative period can be important questions for medicines such as oral contraceptives, oral hypoglycaemics and antihypertensive therapy. Clinical pharmacists can advise on the appropriate action to be taken, which may include temporarily omitting some medicines and/or using short-term alternatives [64].

Accurate documentation of drug allergies and intolerances, important in any area of pharmacy practice, is especially significant for patients undergoing surgery and requiring anaesthesia. Clinical pharmacists also give advice on subjects such as appropriate antibiotic and thromboembolic prophylaxis and postoperative pain control.

To help ensure that hospital beds and other facilities are used in the most efficient manner, it is essential that admission and discharge procedures run smoothly, particularly for planned surgery. This can involve clinical pharmacist attendance at preadmission clinics, comprehensive medication history taking, the extensive use of PODs and self-medication schemes and, more recently, pharmacist prescribing of medication for discharge [65].

HIV/AIDS

Human immunodeficiency virus (HIV)-infected patients are now living longer, the number of treatment options available is constantly expanding and patient expectations and knowledge of medicines are often much greater than in other areas of clinical practice [66]. Specialist clinical pharmacist posts were initially established to provide clinicians and managers with detailed information to ensure safe, effective and economic use of the drugs available for patients with HIV/acquired immunodeficiency syndrome (AIDS). Clinical pharmacy input has since expanded considerably. Services include the provision of detailed education and counselling to help patients cope with the complicated treatment regimens used and identification and management of side-effects and ADRs, common problems with medicines used to treat HIV/AIDS.

The constant addition of new drugs means that frequent amendments to clinical guidelines and treatment protocols are required and the management of medicines used in clinical trials also forms a significant part of many pharmacists' workload. Finally, pharmacist input into good-quality financial management helps to ensure that patients with HIV/AIDS can be treated with medicines in a cost-effective manner to maximise the benefits that can be achieved with the limited resources available.

Critical and intensive care units and theatres

Critical and intensive care medicine has evolved into a major multidisciplinary area of clinical practice and clinical pharmacists have become increasingly integrated into this complex discipline. Whilst many of the responsibilities of clinical pharmacists are not specific to critical and intensive care, the nature of the patients being treated and the complexity of the treatment being given make things more difficult. Table 7.2 details these [67].

Specialist clinical pharmacists can have detailed knowledge and experience in the care given in critical and intensive care units. However, close liaison with other pharmacy colleagues in addition to medical, nursing and other health care staff is also paramount, particularly in relation to medicines information and aseptic dispensing services.

The role of the clinical pharmacist in operating theatres is less well established in the UK, although it is being developed in some centres as the helpful contribution that the clinical pharmacist can make is recognised. In addition to providing advice on rational drug use, health and safety issues and minimising drug wastage are key activities [68].

Nutrition

Pharmacy departments have for many years provided a core input to the provision of parenteral nutrition. Intravenous nutrition services are an example *par excellence* of the multidisciplinary teamwork involving physicians, surgeons, nurses, dietitians and pharmacists working together to deliver care to meet the needs of individual patients.

Table 7.2   The issues for critical care pharmacists

Patients frequently have multiorgan failure, affecting drug distribution, metabolism and elimination
Multiple drug use significantly increases the risk of interactions
Difficulties in identifying adverse drug reactions in patients on multiple drug therapies
The need to ensure the correct method of administration coupled with the frequent physical and chemical incompatibilities
The increased incidence of medical emergencies
Medicines may need to be given outside their licensed recommendations
The need for 24-hour availability of clinical pharmacy input

The siting of aseptic dispensaries in acute hospitals has led to the pharmaceutical input to selection of nutrients, formulation and preparation of compounded solutions that are tailor-made to the needs of, and which can be administered directly to, the patient.

The importance of delivering macronutrients, e.g. amino acids, glucose, fat, electrolytes and water, to patients is crucial for repleting daily nutritional requirements and meeting the higher needs in hypercatabolic patients. Amino acids must always be given at the same time as the calorie source in order to achieve optimal utilisation into protein and peptides.

Micronutrients, such as trace elements and vitamins and some drugs, can also be incorporated into the regimen. These compounded solutions are referred as intravenous nutrition (IVN) or total parenteral nutrition (TPN). Such solutions are used for premature infants and infants and adults requiring nutritional support where the enteral route is not suitable. Some patients who have gut failure or require an extensive period of gut rest are, if suitable, placed on a home IVN programme. Considerable multidisciplinary support is needed for such patients.

Oncology

Pharmacy departments have also traditionally been involved in the preparation of cytotoxic chemotherapy. As with the IVN solutions described above, this has emanated from the technical support for the preparation of these products but with cytotoxic chemotherapy there has been the additional requirement of health and safety considerations. Again the multidisciplinary approach to care of oncology patients has become a particular feature. This is highlighted in the Cancer Plan and also the National Cancer Standards. Table 7.3 lists the particular contributions that clinical pharmacists can make.

Paediatrics

Pharmaceutical formulation and preparation of medicines suitable for children are still major roles for hospital pharmacy. The risks and high costs associated with intravenous treatment make the clinical input of pharmacists essential components of any aseptic manufacturing and preparation services. Aseptic services are covered in detail in chapter 4.

Near-patient clinical pharmacy services in paediatrics have also become increasingly challenging. For individual patients the pharmacist

Table 7.3 Roles of the clinical pharmacist in oncology

Prescribing regimens

Dose modifications in renal and hepatic disease

Antimicrobial therapy

Nausea and vomiting regimens

Management of anaphylactic shock

Extravasation policies

Palliative care

Education and training

Patient education

Clinical trials

Liaison with primary care

can give specialist advice on many aspects of drug treatment. As the survival rates for premature babies improve, pharmacists are also expected to advise on drug therapy in a new patient population for which there are often few data.

In a wider context, the increased involvement of pharmacists has also resulted in the joint production of specialist paediatric guidelines, protocols and formularies that are now routinely used to help answer the many questions that could not be found in the standard reference sources previously available.

The financial implications of drug therapy are of particular significance in paediatrics. In cases where lifelong treatment is indicated, it will be taken for far longer than by adult patients with the same condition. Also, the lack of dedicated paediatric formulations for many products can potentially result in high levels of waste, so clinical pharmacists working in paediatrics have a major role in medicines budgetary planning and control [69].

Renal services

The need to adjust medication doses in patients with renal impairment has been established for many years. However, major developments in dialysis techniques and the introduction of many new treatment options for renal patients have provided hospital pharmacists with exciting opportunities to make a major contribution to patient care. In addition, the chronic nature of the disease means that patients typically return to hospital at regular intervals, enabling the pharmacist to establish good long-term working relationships.

Pharmacists can be instrumental in helping to establish local treatment guidelines and medicines formularies for the treatment of the renal disease itself, but they also have a major role to play in advising on appropriate drug choice and dose for other conditions that may coexist in a patient with renal disease. This will include establishing the risks and benefits of each treatment option relative to other drugs and will typically require information on the extent of drug removal by the various dialysis techniques employed [70].

Renal patients tend to be prescribed a large number of medicines and the regimens can also be comparatively complicated. Pharmacist advice to medical staff can help to simplify many treatment regimens, making life easier for patients and in some cases reducing costs of treatment or the risk of ADRs. However, patient counselling and education still form a large part of renal pharmacists' workload, to help maximise concordance with prescribed treatment and ensure that patients can achieve the long-term benefits that the medicines can confer [71].

Mental health

Many clinical pharmacy activities within mental health are shared with other areas of pharmacy practice. However, a number of other key factors have contributed to the need for increased clinical pharmacy input [72, 73]:

- the increased risk of suicide in mental health patients not adequately treated
- potential risks associated with the high dose and other unlicensed treatments sometimes prescribed in mental health
- the increasing use of high-cost 'atypical' antipsychotics
- the need for close monitoring of patients on clozapine, an antipsychotic that can affect patients' white cell counts
- dependence and/or misuse of some drug treatments (e.g. benzodiazepines, opiates) or alcohol
- the increasing emphasis on community-based treatment for patients with mental health problems.

Clinical pharmacists in mental health typically work within large multidisciplinary teams and much of their input into patient care is provided during attendance at ward rounds, team meetings and patient case conferences. When patients are going to be treated at home, communication with community-based health care professionals, patient education, organisation of self-medication programmes and provision of compliance aids where necessary are all important roles for the pharmacist to help ensure the success of long-term therapy.

Moving into prescribing

The term 'prescribing' has been a contentious issue for many years when discussing potential roles for the pharmacist. In fact, the terms 'prescribe', 'supply' and 'administer' are often used imprecisely in relation to medicines and have been subject to widespread interpretation [74]. In its simplest form, prescribing can be defined as a single function: communicating medication orders to the patient or to other member of the health care team. However, prescribing is more commonly thought of as part of a complex process consisting of multiple tasks. This can include patient assessment, investigations, diagnosis and follow-up, in addition to prescribing, monitoring and adjusting drug treatment. Although pharmacists are not qualified to undertake all these functions alone, they can certainly participate in the prescribing process as part of the multidisciplinary team.

In 1997, the UK government announced a major review of the arrangements for the prescribing, supply and administration of medicines, led by Dr June Crown, President of the Faculty of Public Health Medicine. Prior to this review, pharmacists and nurses at some UK hospitals had already expanded their clinical role to include authorising the administration of medicines, including prescription-only medicines (POMs), without a doctor being involved in every case, but following locally approved protocols [75]. For example, some hospital pharmacists have extended their roles to include writing orders for patients' discharge medication, based on the inpatient prescription chart [76, 77]. However, by carrying out this transcription the pharmacist is not actually prescribing within the legal definitions, as the original authorisation to supply and administer the medicines was made by a doctor. The first report from the Crown review team in 1998 [78] made recommendations on how these arrangements should operate, originally giving them the term 'group protocols'. The protocols have since been renamed 'patient group directions' and allow the supply and/or administration of POMs in accordance with a written protocol signed by both a doctor and a pharmacist.

The final report on the prescribing, supply and administration of medicines in the UK was published in March 1999 [74]. As widely expected, it proposed that new groups of health care professionals, including pharmacists, would be able to apply for authority to prescribe medicines in specific clinical areas, where this would improve patient care and patient safety could be assured. The report listed a number of factors that led to this conclusion:

- growing expertise in advanced clinical roles in many professions
- an increasing tendency for professionals to work together in multiprofessional teams
- the need for responsibility and accountability for clinical care to be clear and unambiguous
- a growing expectation from patients that they will experience a 'seamless service'
- a growing wish to choose the most convenient pathway through the clinical system in cases where there are equally safe and effective clinical alternatives.

The report recommended that two types of prescriber should be recognised:

- the independent prescriber who is responsible for assessing patients with un-diagnosed conditions and for decisions about the clinical management required, including prescribing. At the time of the report, this included doctors, dentists and certain nurses in respect of a limited list of medicines. Certain other health care professionals could become legally authorised independent prescribers, subject to detailed limitations
- the dependent prescriber who is responsible for the continuing care of patients who have been clinically assessed by an independent prescriber. This continuing care may include prescribing, which is usually informed by clinical guidelines and consistent with individual treatment plans; or continuing established treatment by issuing repeat prescriptions, with the authority to adjust the dose or dosage form according to the patients' needs. There should be provision for regular clinical review by the assessing clinician. The nomenclature has since been amended and this is now referred to as 'supplementary prescribing', not 'dependent prescribing'.

In recognising that prescribing privileges should be extended to pharmacists (and other health care professionals) in the hospital setting, the report is likely to speed up the removal of professional boundaries in the UK. This will require the extensive cooperation of doctors, nurses, pharmacists and other health care professionals. At the time of writing the process of establishing supplementary prescribing is being progressed for pharmacists and nurses.

In a 1998 UK study [79], few hospital doctors and nurses had any experience of prescriptions written by a pharmacist, but all those who did had found it helpful. Many doctors and nurses supported the concept of pharmacist-written prescriptions and pharmacist prescribing in a wide range of scenarios, although a significant number also had reservations. As a relatively new introduction to health care (with the exception of pharmacist input into anticoagulant clinics, described above), there are currently few published data on pharmacist prescribing in the UK, although recent studies have been successful [80, 81]. The common factor contributing to the successes of pharmacist prescribing to date is that the pharmacist does not prescribe and monitor drug treatment in isolation, but does so in collaboration with medical staff who have made the necessary diagnosis. Acceptance of a higher degree of responsibility and provision of comprehensive pharmaceutical care for patients should ensure that pharmacists can contribute to improved patient outcomes [8].

The future

Optimising the use of medicines in hospitals is central to the delivery of high-quality patient care. Medication errors in hospitals are still unacceptably common and medicines continue to become increasingly complex and more costly. The future of medicines management is inextricably linked with clinical pharmacy, with much of the value that pharmacists can add being information provision and monitoring quality.

The 2001 report from the UK Audit Commission's investigation into medicines management in hospitals may well prove to be the catalyst that the profession needs [1]. It also signals to those outside the profession the importance of pharmaceutical services to patient care. The report acknowledged that current evidence supports innovation in many areas of hospital pharmacy practice; Table 7.4 identifies these.

The analytical instruments that were employed by the Audit Commission's review of hospital services together with the performance management of medicines management in NHS hospitals are likely to form the basis for a national continuing monitoring programme for the effectiveness of hospital pharmacy services.

Pharmacy services in the future will need to be designed around the needs of patients, not organisations, integrated with other health care services, designed to make the best use of staff and their skills and take advantage of modern technologies. Although computers can help undertake some of this work, there are limitations to the possible achievements of technology and there is no substitute for direct contact with patients. Clinical pharmacy services in hospital have changed significantly over the last few decades, but reengineering the way in which

Table 7.4   Innovations in practice supported by the Audit Commission [1]

Proactive care on admission

Re-engineering supply through the use of original pack dispensing

Medication review clinics

Better use of pharmacy technicians

Development of proactive clinical pharmacy services

Self-administration of medicines by patients

Pharmacist prescribing

The use of information technology and automation

A number of key roles for hospital pharmacy services of the future were also identified:

- Pharmacist prescribing
- Clinical governance
- Preparing guidelines of clinical care
- Attending ward rounds
- Teaching
- Reviewing whole health economy prescribing
- Running selected clinics
- Medicines information services

patient care is delivered is an ongoing process. Many of the changes are designed to free up hospital pharmacists' time to focus even more on the delivery of clinical care. Despite their limitations, the use of electronic prescribing and automated dispensing systems can help pharmacists to devote more of their time to patient care. Revision and expansion of the pharmacy technician and pharmacy assistant roles also need to play a major part in this strategy.

The long-term vision for clinical pharmacy is a service contributing to a health service that offers patients fast and convenient care, available when they need it, tailored to their individual requirements and delivered to a consistently high standard. Delivering a successful clinical pharmacy service will bring major benefits to patients and pharmacists alike.

References

1.   Audit Commission. *A Spoonful of Sugar – Medicines Management in NHS Hospitals*. London: Audit Commission, 2001.
2.   NHS Executive. *Information for Health, An Information Strategy for a Modern NHS 1998–2005*. London: NHS Executive, 1998.

3. Clucas K, chair. *Pharmacy: A Report to the Nuffield Foundation*. London: Nuffield Foundation, 1986.

4. Cotter S M, Barber N D, McKee M. Professionalisation of hospital pharmacy: the role of clinical pharmacy. *J Soc Admin Pharm* 1994; 11: 57–67.

5. Department of Health. Health Services Management. *The Way Forward for Hospital Pharmaceutical Services*. HC(88)54. London: Department of Health, 1988.

6. Cotter S, Barber N, McKee M. Survey of clinical pharmacy services in United Kingdom National Health Service hospitals. *Am J Hosp Pharm* 1994; 51: 2676–2684.

7. Calvert R T. Clinical pharmacy – a hospital perspective. *Br J Clin Pharmacol* 1998; 47: 231–238.

8. Hepler C D, Strand L M. Opportunities and responsibilities in pharmaceutical care. *Am J Hosp Pharm* 1990; 47: 533–543.

9. Department of Health. *A First Class Service, Quality in the New NHS*. London: The Stationery Office, 1998.

10. Walker R, Bussey R. Assessment of a hospital based clinical pharmacy service. *Pharm J* 1986; 237: 558.

11. Hawkey C, Hodgson S, Norman A *et al*. Effect of reactive pharmacy intervention on quality of hospital prescribing. *BMJ* 1990; 300: 986–990.

12. Jenkins D, Cairns C, Barber N. The quality of written inpatient prescriptions. *Int J Pharm Pract* 1993; 2: 176–179.

13. Bentley A, Green R. Developing pharmacutical services; the nursing view. *Br J Pharm Pract* 1981; 3: 4–9.

14. Cavell G F, Bunn R J, Hodges M. Consultants' views on the developing role of the hospital pharmacist. *Pharm J* 1987; 239: 100–102.

15. Fletcher P, Barber N. The pharmacist's contribution to clinicians' ward rounds: analysis by the stages in the drug use process. *Int J Pharm Pract* 1995; 3: 241–244.

16. Cairns C J, Prior F G R. The clinical pharmacist: a study of his hospital involvement. *Pharm J* 1983; 320: 16–18.

17. Trewin V F, Town R. Pharmacist effectiveness at case conferences. *Br J Pharm Pract* 1986; 8: 298–304.

18. Department of Health. *Building a Safer NHS for Patients. Implementing an Organisation with a Memory*. London: Department of Health, 2001.

19. Winstanley P, Irvin L, Smith J *et al*. Adverse drug reactions: a hospital pharmacy-based reporting scheme. *Br J Clin Pharmacol* 1989; 28: 113–116.

20. Lee A, Bateman D N, Edwards C *et al*. Reporting of adverse drug reactions by hospital pharmacists: pilot scheme. *BMJ* 1997; 315: 519.

21. Green C, Mottram D, Rowe P, Brown A. Adverse drug reaction monitoring by United Kingdom hospital pharmacy departments: impact of the introduction of 'yellow card' reporting for pharmacists. *Int J Pharm Pract* 1999; 7: 238–246.

22. Dodds L. An objective assessment of the role of the pharmacist in medication and compliance history taking. *Br J Pharm Pract* 1982; 4: 12–24.

23. Hebron B, Jay C. Pharmaceutical care for patients undergoing elective ENT surgery. *Pharm J* 1998; 260: 65–66.

24. Hick H, Deady P, Wright D, Silcock J. The impact of the pharmacist on an elective general surgery pre-admission clinic. *Pharm World Sci* 2001; 23: 65–69.

25. Department of Health. *Pharmacy in the Future – Implementing the NHS Plan*. London: Department of Health, 2000.

26. Bloom B S. Daily regimen and compliance with treatment. *BMJ* 2001; 323: 647.

27. Royal Pharmaceutical Society of Great Britain. *From Compliance to Concordance: Towards Shared Goals in Medicine Taking*. London: RPSGB, 1997.

28. Varma S, McElnay J C, Hughes C M *et al*. Pharmaceutical care of patients with congestive heart failure: interventions and outcomes. *Pharmacotherapy* 1999; 19: 860–869.

29. Johnston M, Clarke A, Mundy K *et al*. Facilitating comprehension of discharge medication in elderly patients. *Age Ageing* 1986; 15: 304–306.

30. Goodyer L, Miskelly F, Milligan P. Does encouraging good compliance improve patients' clinical condition in heart failure? *Br J Clin Pract* 1995; 49: 173–176.

31. Al-Eidan F A, McElnay J C, Scott M G, McConnell J B. Management of *Helicobacter pylori* eradication – the influence of structured counselling and follow-up. *Br J Clin Pharmacol* 2002; 53: 163–171.

32. Sandler D, Mitchell J, Fellows A, Garner S. Is an information booklet for patients leaving hospital helpful and useful? *BMJ* 1989; 298: 870–874.

33. McElnay J, Scott M, Armstrong A, Stanford C. Audiovisual demonstration for patient counselling in the use of pressurised aerosol bronchodilator inhalers. *J Clin Pharm Ther* 1989; 14: 135–144.

34. Daly M, Jones S. Preliminary assessment of a computerised counselling program for asthmatic children. *Pharm J* 1991; 247: 206–208.

35. Raynor D, Booth T, Blenkinsopp A. Effects of computer generated reminder charts on patients' compliance with drug regimens. *BMJ* 1993; 306: 1158–1161.

36. Woloshin S, Schwartz L M, Tremmel J, Welch H G. Direct-to-consumer advertisements for prescription drugs: what are Americans being sold? *Lancet* 2001; 358: 1141–1146.

37. Wood S I, Calvert R T, Acomb C, Kay L. A self-medication scheme for elderly patients improves compliance with their medication regimens *Int J Pharm Pract* 1992; 1: 240–241.

38. Lowe C J, Raynor D K, Courtney E A *et al*. Effects of a self-medication programme on knowledge of drugs and compliance with treatment in elderly patients. *BMJ* 1995; 310: 1229–1231.

39. Bourne J, Farrar K, Fitzpatrick R. Practical involvement in therapeutic drug monitoring. *Pharm J* 1985; 234: 530–531.

40. Brown A. Establishment of a pharmacy-run TDM service. *Br J Pharm Pract* 1986; 8: 154–159.

41. Campbell D. A clinical pharmacokinetics service. *Hosp Pharm* 1999; 6: 206–208.

42. Anonymous. Postgraduate education for hospital pharmacists. *Pharm J* 1978; 220: 525–526.

43. Noyce P, Hibberd A. Launch of the London MSc in Clinical Pharmacy. *Pharm J* 1980; 225: 4733–4734.

44. Baker J. Seventeen years experience of a voluntary based drug rationalisation program in hospital. *BMJ* 1988; 297: 465–469.

45. *Moving to Audit: What Every Pharmacist Needs to Know about Professional Audit.* Dundee: The Postgraduate Office, Ninewells Hospital and Medical School, 1993.

46. Davies H T O. Developing effective clinical audit. *Hosp Med* 1999; 60: 748–750.

47. Teasdale S. The future of clinical audit: learning to work together. *BMJ* 1996; 313: 574.

48. Booth C. Pharmacist-managed anticoagulation clinics: a review. *Pharm J* 1998; 261: 623–625.

49. Boddy C. Pharmacist involvement with warfarin dosing for inpatients. *Pharm World Sci* 2001; 23: 31–35.

50. Dean J, Acomb J. A pharmacist managed lithium clinic. *Hosp Pharm* 1995; 2: 150–152.

51. Jones S, Pritchard M, Grout C *et al.* A rheumatology drug monitoring clinic. *Pharm J* 1999; 263: 25.

52. Williams H. Pharmacist-led lipid management clinic. *Pharm J* 1999; 263: 26.

53. Brown J, Brown D. Pharmaceutical care at the primary–secondary interface in Portsmouth and South East Hampshire. *Pharm J* 1997; 258: 280–284.

54. Ashby N, Taylor D. Patient-controlled analgesia and the hospital pharmacist. *Hosp Pharm* 1994; 1: 38–41.

55. Mitchell K, Clarke C. The provision of pharmaceutical care to hospice patients. *Pharm J* 1996; 256: 352–353.

56. Needham D. Improving palliative care in the community. *Pharm J* 1999; 263: 21.

57. Colaluca A, Glet R, Smith D *et al.* In-patient counselling – a technician's role. *Br J Pharm Pract* 1988; 10: 334–340.

58. Dosaj R, Mistry R. The pharmacy technician in clinical services. *Hosp Pharm* 1998; 5: 26–28.

59. Edwards L. The role of the directorate liaison technician. *Hosp Pharm* 2001; 8: 115–116.

60. Department of Health. *Medicines and Older People. Implementing Medicines-related Aspects of the NSF for Older People.* London: Department of Health, 2001.

61. Cannon J, Hughes C. Pharmaceutical care provision to elderly patients: an assessment of its impact on compliance and discharge medication changes. *Eur Hosp Pharm* 1999; 5: 102–105.

62. Foster P. Pharmacy services to a medical admission ward. *Pharm J* 1995; 254: 656–657.

63. Scott M G, Stanford C, Nicholls D *et al.* Reduction of ward drug costs by clinical pharmacist involvement. *Pharm J* 1987; 239: 73–79.

64. Smith H. Pharmacist involvement in a surgical preadmission clinic improves the quality of patient care. *Pharm J* 1997; 259: 902.

65. Dobrzanski S, Reidy F. The pharmacist as a discharge medication planner in surgical patients. *Pharm J* 1993; 250: HS53–HS56.

66. Weston R. The changing role of the HIV pharmacist – how can we influence drug prescribing and expenditure? *Hosp Pharm* 1996; 3: 83–85.

67. Sani M, Bihari D. The specialist critical care pharmacist. *Hosp Pharm* 1995; 2: 37–39.

68. Davis S. The directorate pharmacist for operating theatres. *Hosp Pharm* 1998; 5: 127–130.

69. Pilkington K. The role of the paediatric pharmacist. *Hosp Pharm* 1994; 1: 42–44.

70. Maclean D. Defining a niche for the renal pharmacist. *Hosp Pharm* 1994; 1: 20–22.

71. Morlidge C. Pharmacist-run renal medication review clinics. *Br J Renal Med* 2001; 6: 25–26.

72. Cloete B, Heath P. Pharmacist participation in a psychiatric consultant ward round. *Pharm J* 1987; 238: 42–43.

73. Kettle J, Downie G, Palin A. Pharmaceutical care activities within a mental health team. *Pharm J* 1996; 257: 814–816.

74. Department of Health. *Review of Prescribing, Supply and Administration of Medicines. Final Report (Crown Report)*. London: Department of Health, 1999.

75. *Medicines, Ethics and Practice. A Guide for Pharmacists*, 26th edn. London: Royal Pharmaceutical Society of Great Britain, 2002.

76. Culshaw M, Dawes S. Assessing the value of a discharge pharmacist. *Pharm Manage* 1998; 14: 22–23.

77. Oliver S, Ashwell S. Pharmacists prescribing take home medication. *Pharm J* 2000; 265: 22.

78. NHS Executive. *A Report on the Supply and Administration of Medicines under Group Protocols*. HSC 1998/051. Leeds: Department of Health, 1998.

79. Child D, Hirsch C, Berry M. Health care professionals' views on hospital pharmacist prescribing in the United Kingdom. *Int J Pharm Pract* 1998; 6: 159–169.

80. Hughes D, Kinnear A, Macintyre J, Pacciti L. Collaborative medicines management: pharmacist prescribing. *Pharm J* 1999; 263: 172.

81. Woolfrey S, Dean C, Hall H. Hospital pharmacist prescribing: a pilot study. *Pharm J* 2000; 265: 97–99.

Further reading

Audit Commission. *A Spoonful of Sugar – Medicines Management in NHS Hospitals*. London: The Audit Commission, 2001.

Department of Health (1999). *Review of Prescribing, Supply and Administration of Medicines. Final Report*. London: Department of Health, 1999. www.doh.gov.uk/prescrib.htm (accessed 10 February 2002).

Department of Health (2000). *Pharmacy in the Future – Implementing the NHS Plan*. London: Department of Health, 2000. www.doh.gov.uk/pharmacyfuture/ (accessed 10 February 2002).

Department of Health (2001). *Building a Safer NHS for Patients. Implementing an Organisation with a Memory*. London: Department of Health, 2001. www.doh.gov.uk/buildsafenhs (accessed 10 February 2002).

8

Strategic medicines management

Ray Fitzpatrick

Medicines are central to most health care interventions and in hospital particularly, since nearly every admission involves the use of a medicine. However, the use of medicines carries risk, both clinically and financially.

Clinical risk

- All medicines are potentially poisons: there are over 1000 deaths per year due to medication errors or adverse events [1].
- Patients are getting older and sicker.
- More medicines are used per patient than ever before.

In relation to the last point, the average number of prescriptions in the community per head of population per year was 8.2 in 1990, but rose to 11 in 2000. However, the over-65 age group received on average 26.5 prescription items per head of population per year in 2000 [2].

Financial risk

- The National Health Service (NHS) spends over £6 billion p.a. on medicines [2].
- There are multifactorial influences on prescribing.
- Some of the drivers for prescribing are outside the NHS, for example, the pharmaceutical industry, and Royal College guidelines.

Therefore, medicines management can be seen as risk management. Chapter 7 gave the Audit Commission definition of medicines management in hospitals – encompassing all aspects of medicine use, influencing the availability and policies on medicines at an organisational level as well as the prescription, use and administration of medicines at an individual patient level. This chapter will focus on the strategic elements of this definition, which are centred around influencing the availability of medicines, the policies on the use of medicines within a hospital, as well as influencing prescribers.

History

The hospital pharmacist's role in medicines management was recognised as long ago as 1955 in the Linstead Report on hospital pharmacy [3]. In this report the role of the hospital pharmacy included:

- to assist in the development of new methods of treatment
- to promote economy in the use of medical supplies
- to assist in efficient prescribing by advising upon the nature and properties of medicaments, and selection of the most suitable substances and the form in which they should be prescribed.

These principles hold true today as they did then, particularly as the range and complexity of medicines have increased enormously. In the intervening years milestone reports such as the Nuffield Report in 1986 [4], the Department of Health (DoH) circular on clinical pharmacy in 1988 [5], and *Pharmacy in the Future* in 2000 [6] reinforced the role of the hospital pharmacist at the centre of medicines management.

Although systems to manage prescribing have a longer history in hospital than in primary care, more attention has focused on primary care with more central initiatives (for example, prescribing analyses and cost (PACT) data, district health authority pharmaceutical advisers and general practice prescribing incentive schemes). This is not surprising since 80% of NHS expenditure on medicines is in primary care.

Prescribing costs have risen significantly in primary care, as shown in Figure 8.1. However, expenditure in secondary care has been growing at a rate of approximately 10% p.a., and stood at just under £1.5bn p.a. in 1999/2000 [1]. It is for these reasons that attention is now being focused on systems for managing medicines in hospital.

Performance management framework

In 2001 the DoH issued a framework for medicines management to all acute trusts [7]. This framework identified six key domains where trusts should have robust systems in place to manage medicines. These were:

1. Senior management awareness and involvement
2. Information and financial issues

3.   Medicines policy management, including the introduction of new drugs
4.   Procurement of medicines
5.   Primary–secondary care interface
6.   Influencing prescribers.

As part of this initiative hospitals had to undertake a self-assessment of where they were in relation to each of these domains. Analysis of results for one NHS region is shown in Figure 8.2. This demonstrates that most trusts have robust systems in relation to procurement of medicines, influencing prescribers, and interfacing with primary care. However,

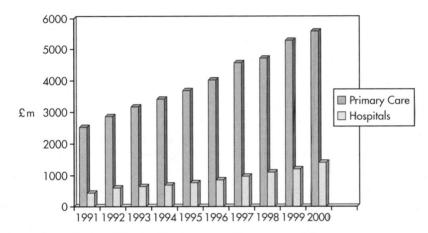

Figure 8.1   National Health Service expenditure on medicines.

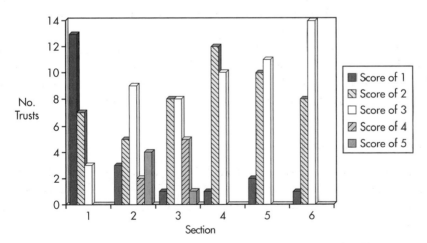

Figure 8.2   Results of Department of Health Medicines Framework self-assessment: West Midlands. A score of 5 shows excellent performance.

systems are less well developed in relation to senior management awareness of prescribing issues, and information on prescribing. It also shows
wide variation in the development of systems for the introduction of
new medicines. A similar pattern is seen across all regions in
England [8].

This initiative has recently been supplemented by the publication
of the Audit Commission report on medicines management in hospital
which makes a number of far-reaching recommendations as well as
raising the profile of medicines management and the role of the hospital
pharmacist [1].

Strategic medicines management in practice

In describing various approaches to implementing strategic medicines
management in practice, it is appropriate to discuss the issue in the
context of the DoH framework, which identified the six principal
domains described above.

Senior management awareness of prescribing issues

Any medicines management system will only succeed if those implementing it, primarily hospital pharmacists, have the support of the most
senior management in the organisation. This requires the trust management board to be fully aware of prescribing issues including expenditure
trends, risks and cost pressures. It is clear from the self-assessment
(Figure 8.2) that this is not well developed in most hospitals. However,
there is evidence in the literature of initiatives where there are regular
prescribing reports presented to the trust management board [9]. An
example of the format of such a report is shown in Table 8.1. This not
only highlights the trust's overall medicines expenditure against budget,
but also individual clinical divisions or directorates (see section on
information and financial issues, below, for details about clinical directorate structure).

This approach focuses management attention on areas where there
may be problems and ensures that clinical directors or heads of division
keep prescribing high on their agenda. What is not shown in Table 8.1
is the detailed narrative describing particular prescribing issues or initiatives in each clinical directorate or division.

This type of prescribing report can also keep the board informed of
decisions of prescribing committees such as the drug and therapeutics
(D&T) committee and also inform performance review meetings

Table 8.1 North Staffordshire hospital trust pharmacy directorate: quarterly drug expenditure management report second quarter July–September 2000

Division	Budget £000k	Actual £000k	Variance £000k	%
Anaesthesia and surgery	807	841	34	4.2
Central	9	9	0	0.0
Clinical support services	106	99	(7)	(6.6)
Locomotor	213	208	(5)	(2.4)
Medicine	957	954	(3)	(0.3)
Specialised services	948	967	19	2.0
Women's and children's	351	322	(29)	(8.3)
Trust total	3391	3400	9	0.27

Drug and Therapeutics Committee

The Drug and Therapeutics Committee considered the following applications for inclusion in the District Formulary on 12 September.

- Fosphenytoin for epilepsy: application made by Dr S Ellis – rejected
- Mometasone for rhinitis: application made by Mr P Wilson – rejected
- Latanoprost for glaucoma: application made by Mr T Gillow – approved.
  For use as a second-line agent, treatment should be initiated by an ophthalmologist. Prescribing should then be transferred to the General Practitioner via a shared-care agreement.

The following applications will be considered on 14 November 2000.

- Cetirizine for urticaria: application made by Dr B Tan
- Bicalutamide for prostate cancer: application made by Mr Liu

Medicines Management Group

The Medicines Management Group reviewed the use of leflunomide and infliximab in the treatment of rheumatoid arthritis on 27 June. The group supported the use of these agents subject to the identification of additional funding. In conjunction with the rheumatologists, business cases will be submitted to the health authority to support the prescribing of leflunomide and infliximab in rheumatoid arthritis.

between the Chief Executive and clinical directors or heads of division/directorate.

As well as highlighting prescribing, these reports also maintain the profile of the hospital pharmacy and the hospital pharmacist's role in medicines management. This approach is one of the key recommendations of the Audit Commission [1].

Information and financial issues

Clearly, if senior management is to be aware of prescribing issues, there needs to be a robust system for collating and reporting information on medicines usage. All hospital pharmacies have computerised stock control systems for medicines. However, these systems are designed around purchasing and stock control, and not producing prescribing reports. Therefore, whilst pharmacy computer systems can provide details on medicines expenditure, obtaining detailed prescribing reports on medicine usage can prove problematic. Some pharmacy computer systems are flexible enough to enable prescribing reports to be produced, but not all systems can be interrogated easily. The fact that there are a variety of commercial systems being used with no common identifier for medicines was highlighted as a problem in a project run by the National Prescribing Centre. This aimed to collect detailed prescribing information routinely from a cohort of hospitals. The results of this pilot project showed some interesting trends, but it proved impossible to roll out across the whole of the NHS because of the above problems [10].

Computerised prescribing linked with electronic patient records will alleviate this problem and provide better information on hospital prescribing patterns, since usage data can be linked to individual patients and diagnosis. More importantly, where computerised prescribing has been implemented, it has delivered significant improvements in the quality of patient care [11]. The NHS information for health strategy expected 53% of hospitals to have installed electronic patient records systems (including reporting of results and prescribing) by 2002, and all trusts by 2005 [12].

As discussed earlier, most hospitals are managed on a directorate structure (see chapter 1). Wards or clinical specialities are grouped together as a clinical directorate, with their own budget and management team. The directorate usually has a clinician as clinical director who is supported by a manager, financial accountant and human resources. In large hospitals, these clinical directorates may be grouped into clinical divisions (that is, medicine, surgery, etc.) which are directly accountable and represented on trust management boards. A survey published in 1997 indicated that 77% of drug budgets were devolved to clinical directorates [13].

In order to support effective medicines management, the key elements of financial and information systems should include:

- expenditure data for the trust as a whole broken down by division/directorate
- drug budgets set at directorate/divisional level
- a system to identify future cost pressures (such as implementing National Institute for Clinical Excellence (NICE) guidance) which can be fed into the commissioning process
- medicines usage data which can be matched with activity (for example, finished consultant episodes or FCEs).

Having a good system for collecting and reporting information on pre-scribing is not only important to help manage the financial risks around medicines, but also the clinical risk. The latter is highlighted by increasing concerns in relation to the emergence of resistance to antibiotics, particularly as a survey of hospital prescribing identified treatment of infections as the highest cost therapeutic area for both inpatients and outpatients [14–16].

The introduction of new drugs, and medicines policy management

Hospitals have a long history of developing systems to manage the introduction of new medicines. However, Figure 8.2 indicates that there is variability in the level of sophistication of these systems. The corner-stones of any system to manage the introduction of new medicines are the hospital formulary and the D&T committee.

Formularies

Hospital formularies can either be a published list of available medi-cines or a list together with prescribing information. In some cases the formulary may not even be published, but is what is available from the hospital pharmacy. A view many hospitals take is that prescribing information is contained in the *British National Formulary*, and the purpose of a formulary is to inform the prescribing doctor what medi-cines are available. Historically formularies have been applied to junior doctors, but more senior doctors, such as consultants, have been allowed to prescribe outside this restricted list. However, with increased management control, rising drug expenditure and the advent of clinical governance, some hospital formularies have been applied rig-orously to all grades of staff, including consultants [9]. Clearly, when implementing such a policy it is necessary to make arrangements for 'the exceptional clinical situation', since a limited range of medicines may not be sufficient to cover every clinical situation. In my own hos-pital we operate such a policy, and consultants may only prescribe outside the formulary with the prior authorisation of the consultant's clinical director.

Deciding the content of the formulary is usually the responsibil-ity of the D&T committee. It is important that such decisions are evi-dence-based and transparent if the formulary is to improve prescribing and be owned by prescribers. When considering the evidence for new medicines, a number of questions need to be addressed:

- What is the safety profile of the medicine? Is it better or worse than existing medicines? Clearly an application would fail if the new medicine had significantly more side-effects. Is the new medicine a black triangle medicine? This may require a more cautious approach.
- What is the efficacy of the new medicine? Is it better than what is already available? Often improved benefits are marginal and need to be balanced against cost.
- Finally what is the cost? Does the medicine offer marginal benefits at an increased cost, or is it revenue-neutral? Is it exactly the same as existing medicines but less expensive? Hospitals must consider primary care costs if patients will be treated with the medicine chronically in primary care. This is to avoid 'loss-leading', where a pharmaceutical company sets the price in hospital artificially low in order to get a drug used, but the drug is very expensive in primary care. Thus overall the new medicine costs the NHS more, since, as discussed previously, 80% of prescribing costs are in primary care.

In order to inform formulary decisions, the published evidence about the new medicine should be reviewed by someone with critical appraisal skills. This is often a medicines information pharmacist or, in larger hospitals, a formulary pharmacist.

Formularies are an effective way of controlling the introduction of new medicines in hospital, because the hospital pharmacy controls the medicines supply chain. However, in primary care, formularies can only be advisory, since the suppliers (the community pharmacy) are independent contractors. As primary care trusts emerge, they will undoubtedly be able to exert more influence over general practitioners and community pharmacies.

The Audit Commission has advised hospital trust boards to agree formularies which are linked to clinical guidelines and NICE guidance. This concept is further developed under the section dealing with influencing prescribers, below.

D&T committees

D&T committees have been established in most hospitals in the UK for many years, and their role in facilitating the development of formularies was endorsed in the DoH health circular HC(88)54 in the late 1980s [5]. In a survey of hospitals in 1994, 97% indicated they had a D&T committee [13]. The results of the Medicines Management Framework self-assessment indicate that this is likely to be 100% now. D&T committees are a multidisciplinary group reporting to the chief executive, medical director or management board and their remit is to look at prescribing issues in the trust.

Membership of the D&T committee varies from hospital to hospital, but usually includes clinicians representing clinical divisions or directorates, the chief pharmacist, a second pharmacist (medicines information or formulary pharmacist), a junior doctor, a microbiologist, a nursing representative, a general practitioner, health authority pharmaceutical adviser and a finance officer.

The role of the D&T committee tends to cover a range of issues related to prescribing and medicines policy, such as:

- oversee the content and implementation of the hospital formulary
- approve prescribing policies (e.g. antibiotics policies)
- approve prescription documentation
- advise the trust on the impact of new medicines
- approve shared-care protocols
- approve initiatives to support cost-effective prescribing (e.g. therapeutic substitution by pharmacists)
- review patient group directives.

The difficulty D&T committees often face is that the evidence may support the introduction of a new medicine, but the costs may be so high that there is an affordability problem. For medicines used across the whole health economy (primary and secondary care), sharing the costs may solve the problem, since the overall drug budget across a whole health economy will be in the tens of millions of pounds. It is for this reason that the involvement of primary care colleagues in hospital D&T committees is important. However, where a new medicine has a potentially high cost, either because it has a high acquisition cost or high usage (or both) and will only be used in the hospital, affordability will be a major issue. In this case the D&T committee, having reviewed the evidence and supported the introduction of a new medicine, may not authorise inclusion in the formulary until a source of funding can be identified. The new medicine may release resources within the hospital which could fund its use, or the hospital may have a drug budget reserve for such in-year pressures. Alternatively a business case may need to be developed and submitted for inclusion in the annual commissioning process. In the latter case, some hospitals have created a smaller executive group to review applications for new high-cost medicines and develop business cases or to allocate funds for such developments [17, 18].

D&T committees have played an important role in controlling the introduction of new medicines and managing medicines policies for over

30 years. With the changes in the NHS of April 2002, there is a need to have much closer working relationships with other prescribing groups across the whole health economy if there is to be a joined-up approach to effective medicines management.

Procurement of medicines

This is such an important subject in controlling the costs of medicines in hospitals that a separate chapter (chapter 2) is devoted to it. From a strategic medicines management perspective, a key issue is that there is a good interface between procurement of medicines and the other elements of a hospital medicines management system. Prescribing policies should inform purchasing decisions and vice versa. Hospitals should avoid negatively loss-leading into primary care, and, as described below, they should be actively working with primary care to reduce the overall cost of prescribing.

The primary–secondary care interface

The interface between primary and secondary care is becoming increasingly important. In the 1980s and early 1990s when hospital drug budgets were cash-limited but general practice drug budgets were not, hospital clinicians commencing patients on expensive new medicines continued in primary care did not present many problems. It is estimated that although hospital prescribing costs represent only 20% of the total NHS expenditure on medicines, they significantly influence the prescribing in primary care. With the establishment of unified budgets across the whole health economy in the late 1990s, primary care drug budgets were also cash-limited and tensions developed across the interface. Since the late 1990s legislative constraints have been removed and this allows movement of resources for prescribing across the primary/secondary care continuum. Thus, where good working relationships exist, it is possible for purchasing decisions to be made in hospital which positively benefit primary care, and for primary care drug budgets to underwrite any excess cost to the hospital.

District prescribing groups emerged in an attempt to harmonise policies across general practice and between primary and secondary care. With the development of primary care groups and primary care trusts (see chapter 1), it is more important than ever that there is a cohesive approach to managing medicines. Key issues in this relationship are:

- adequate cross-representation on primary care and secondary care prescribing committees
- harmonisation of primary and secondary care formularies
- systems to agree shared-care arrangements
- systems to agree policies to facilitate seamless patient care across the secondary/primary care continuum (e.g. use of patient packs on discharge from hospital).

As discussed in a preceding section, the involvement of primary care in hospital D&T committees is very important. However, the involvement of hospital colleagues in district prescribing groups is just as important. Membership of district prescribing groups usually includes general practitioners, prescribing leads from relevant primary care organisations, health authority pharmaceutical adviser, primary care formulary pharmacist (if one exists), chair of the hospital D&T committee and the hospital chief pharmacist.

The district prescribing committee generally has the following roles:

- oversee the development and implementation of a district-wide primary care formulary
- approve shared-care guidelines
- agree prescribing policies across primary care
- discuss hospital prescribing policies which impact on primary care.

It is clear that district prescribing committees mirror hospital D&T committees, and the challenge is to ensure harmonisation of the work of both groups.

Shared-care agreements

One of the key roles of a district prescribing committee is to take overall responsibility for shared-care agreements. These are protocols for high-technology, complex and often expensive medicines which are commenced in hospital by specialist consultants, but where treatment needs to be continued in primary care. Often general practitioners are uneasy about taking on the prescribing responsibility for highly complex medicines of which they have little experience. However, it is usually impractical for the patient to be seen at the hospital just to receive a repeat prescription. In these cases a shared-care agreement is developed which informs the general practitioner about the medicine, and gives advice, particularly on routine monitoring.

In such agreements the hospital clinician initiates treatment until the patient is stable, and monitors the patient at regular intervals while the general practitioner maintains the patient on treatment in the usual way.

Shared-care agreements should include the following elements:

- **Patient-specific.** Agreements should be patient-specific and encompass all aspects relevant to a particular patient. However, it is recognised that a medicine-specific template may be used which is individualised for the patient.
- **A reasonably predictable clinical situation.** Clinical responsibility should be considered for transfer to primary care only where it is agreed that the patient's clinical condition is stable or predictable.
- **Willing and informed consent of all parties.** Patients, carers and doctors should all consent to a shared-care agreement.
- **Definition of responsibility.** A shared-care agreement should clearly identify the areas of care for which each partner has responsibility.
- **Communication.** An agreement should include a telephone, fax or e-mail contact point in case problems arise.
- **Clinical summary.** This should include a brief overview of the disease and more detailed information on the treatment being transferred for which each partner has managerial and clinical responsibility. This should include the product's licensed indications, therapeutic classification, dose, route of administration, adverse events, monitoring requirements and responsibilities, clinically relevant drug interactions and their management, storage and peer-reviewed references for the product usage.
- **Training.** Where additional training for general practitioners and their staff is necessary, this should be identified and arranged by the referring specialist.

Influencing prescribers

Influencing prescribers occurs at two levels: corporate level and individual level.

Influencing prescribing at a corporate level

This starts with increasing senior management awareness of prescribing issues, as described earlier in this chapter. This influences prescribers in two ways: firstly by management pressure through the divisional/directorate structure and secondly as clinicians are within the management of the hospital. However, one of the most effective ways of influencing prescribing is through the clinical directorate structure. This approach was proposed in the early 1990s, and has resulted in the establishment of directorate pharmacists [19, 20]. These pharmacists are employed by the pharmacy to provide prescribing advice at clinical directorate level. The pharmacist reviews the prescribing trends within a directorate and identifies areas where improvements in prescribing practice can be made. The concept is that the clinical directorate management team agrees a prescribing policy which is then implemented through meetings with senior clinicians, bulletins and clinical pharmacists at ward level. Often initiatives are aimed at improving economy in prescribing and include promoting alternative therapeutic options (that is, reducing the use of unnecessary intravenous antibiotics, or promoting a particular proton pump inhibitor) [9].

Since much of the work at directorate level involves reviewing medicines usage data and producing graphical representation of prescribing trends, pharmacy technicians are now being employed to support directorate pharmacists [21].

Printed bulletins have long been a tool used by pharmacy departments to deliver prescribing messages to doctors across a clinical speciality or whole hospital. However, these bulletins are designed around a particular medicine or group of medicines, and these messages have to be repeated when there is a changeover of medical staff. An alternative approach is to incorporate therapeutic messages as part of clinical guidelines, which are designed around a particular disease state. The advantage is that the prescribing message is an integral part of the care pathway the doctor will be using rather than a separate guideline. This approach has been developed by a consortium of hospitals in the Midlands, which produced a book of clinical guidelines covering a range of disease states in adult acute medicine. An example of a typical guideline incorporating prescribing advice is shown in Figure 8.3. The guideline is produced by one hospital on behalf of the consortium, but each hospital can individualise the guideline if necessary [22].

Influencing individual prescribers

The role of the clinical pharmacist is to promote the safe, rational and cost-effective use of medicines. Clinical pharmacists started to emerge in the 1970s, but it was not until 1988 that their role was formally recognised by the DoH [5]. Often the term 'ward pharmacist' is used to describe pharmacists involved in clinical activities. Initially ward pharmacists visited wards to initiate supplies of non-stock medicines, and clinical pharmacists attended consultant ward rounds to advise on prescribing. However, today the two terms are synonymous, since most of

COMMUNITY ACQUIRED PNEUMONIA • 1/3

RECOGNITION AND ASSESSMENT

Treat as pneumonia if symptoms and signs below plus new unexplained chest x-ray shadowing and the illness is the primary clinical problem

Symptoms

● Malaise, fever, rigors
● Vomiting, diarrhoea
● Confusion (especially in the elderly)
● Dyspnoea, cough
● Sputum (may be blood-stained, viscid and difficult to expectorate)
● Pleuritic pain

Signs

● High fever (often absent in the elderly)
● Tachycardia
● Tachypnoea
● Localized crackles
● Bronchial breathing (in about one third of hospital admissions)
● Chest signs may be absent or masked by other respiratory signs (eg COPD, CCF)

Enquire about pet birds (psittacosis, chlamydia) and recent hotel residence away from home (legionellosis)

Investigations

● Chest x-ray
● Arterial blood gases
● FBC, biochemical screen, CRP
● Microbiology:

Sputum - inspection, microscopy, culture and sensitivity

Blood - cultures: in the seriously ill, serology for atypical organisms (influenza A and B, *Coxiella burnetii, Chlamydia psittaci, Mycoplasma pneumoniae, Legionella pneumophila*)

Urine - in the seriously ill, legionella antigen

Indicators for severity: mental confusion multilobar involvement, respiratory failure, respiratory rate > 30/min, diastolic blood pressure < 60 mm Hg, wbc low (< 4 x 10⁹/l) or very high (> 20 x 10⁹/l), serum urea > 7 mmol/l, serum albumin < 35 g/l

Differential Diagnosis

● Pulmonary thromboembolism
● Lung cancer
● Left ventricular failure

IMMEDIATE TREATMENT

Supportive

● Oxygen to maintain arterial PaO_2 > 8 kPa

In patients with COPD, start with 24% by Ventimask or 1 L/min via nasal prongs and watch for signs of CO_2 narcosis. See **Respiratory Failure**

● Maintain fluid balance
● Adequate analgesia for pleuritic pain: indometacin 25-50 mg orally 8 hrly
● Treat any accompanying airflow obstruction or cardiac failure
● Physiotherapy **only** in patients with copious secretions

Antibiotic Therapy

● Start as soon as diagnosis is made: therapy should **always** cover *Streptococcus pneumoniae*
● Route of administration depends on the severity of illness and likely pathogens
● **Pneumonia of unknown aetiology**

Uncomplicated:

Co-amoxiclav 375 mg orally 8 hrly

In penicillin-allergic patients, use erythromycin 500 mg orally 6 hrly

Figure 8.3 A guideline for managing community-acquired pneumonia.

the supply function has been devolved to pharmacy technicians. Pharmacists influence prescribing by routinely visiting wards to review patients' prescription charts, interact with medical and nursing staff on the wards and, where time allows, attend ward rounds with clinical teams. In reviewing charts, the pharmacist is influencing prescribing

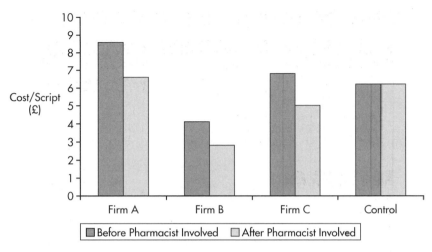

Figure 8.4   Impact of clinical pharmacists on prescribing costs.

retrospectively, whereas at ward rounds the pharmacist is influencing doctors prospectively. Clinical pharmacists have been shown to reduce the prescribing costs of clinical teams significantly, as shown in Figure 8.4. [9]

The role of the clinical pharmacist is described in more detail in chapter 7.

External influences on strategic medicines management in hospitals

NHS reforms

Hospitals do not work in isolation. They have to work in partnership with primary care in order to ensure the safe and effective use of medicines across the primary/secondary care continuum. During the 20th century, when the NHS was formed, hospitals were the main drivers of care and often dictated practice, particularly in relation to prescribing. However, as we entered the 21st century, the emphasis for patient care shifted to primary care. The NHS reforms implemented in April 2002 (see chapter 1) radically changed the health care landscape, and will most certainly impact on prescribing. With the demise of district health authorities, new structures will need to be formed to address issues of prescribing in primary and secondary care.

District prescribing groups are already in place but may need to be reconstituted, with membership to reflect the importance of primary care trusts. A major change will be how funding is secured for new medicines and this reflects the fact that primary care trusts will be undertaking the commissioning of hospital services. There will be an increasing need for evidence-based reviews to support investment in new medicines. Figure 8.5 is a flow chart outlining the route an application for a new medicine in hospital may take in the future.

NICE guidance

Prior to 1999, it was entirely at the discretion of the hospital which new medicine was prescribed in hospital. Where funding a new medicine was an issue, decisions were taken in conjunction with the district health

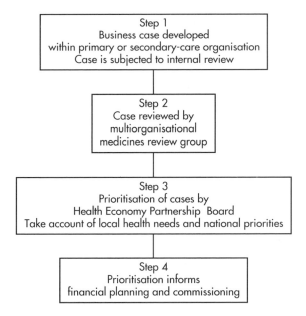

Medicines Review Group
- Critically appraises business cases in relation to evidence, costing/epidemiological assumptions and value for money. Where necessary, challenges/seeks clarification from organisation.
- Has the authority to approve/reject cases before consideration at steps 3 and 4.
- Does not prioritise cases.
- Membership from all primary- and secondary-care organisations with skills to appraise business cases critically for new medicines.

Figure 8.5 The introduction of new medicines not covered by National Institute for Clinical Excellence (NICE) guidance. This applies to new medicines where there are significant resource implications across the whole health economy, or if it affects one organisation only, it cannot be funded internally.

authority. This resulted in variations in availability of new medicines across the whole NHS – so-called 'postcode prescribing'. NICE was established in 1999 with the explicit remit of eliminating postcode prescribing.

The terms of reference for NICE were:

- to reduce inequalities in treatment
- to produce evidence-based guidance on treatments
- to identify new developments which will most improve patient care
- to help protect patients from outdated and inefficient treatments.

In its first 2 years NICE produced over 30 pieces of guidance, most of which cover medicines. Although NICE technology appraisals are called guidance, it is clear that the government does not see this as advisory, but mandatory. Hitherto implementation of NICE guidance has been variable between health authorities, largely due to the enormous resource implications and varying cost pressures on different health authorities. There is now an expectation that commissioning organisations will provide funding to ensure NICE recommendations can be implemented within 3 months of their issue.

Thus, NICE guidance is now obligatory. This will mean that resources will be prioritised for implementing NICE recommendations, estimated at approximately £250m in 2001 [23].

There are three main challenges for hospitals:

1. Develop systems for forward planning as regards the implications of implementing NICE guidance
2. Develop systems for monitoring the implementation of NICE guidance
3. Ensure that new medicines, of proven benefit to the patient but not subject to a NICE recommendation, do not become 'orphan' medicines, because funding has been prioritised for NICE guidance.

In all these challenges the hospital pharmacist has a key role to play. As a result of pharmacists' close working relationship with clinical divisions and directorates, and skills in relation to evidence-based medicine, they can reliably inform the financial planning process. They can also monitor the implementation of NICE guidance as described above in the section on information and financial issues. The hospital pharmacist is an integral part of the D&T committee and medicines management group structures, which will have to champion the introduction of new medicines of proven benefit not covered by NICE guidance.

Conclusion

Strategic medicines management is essentially about influencing prescribing at corporate level, within and between organisations in a health economy. The DoH has set out the key elements of medicines management in hospital. The Audit Commission has reinforced this message and made specific recommendations for improved medicines management in hospitals. This chapter has described various ways in which these concepts can be implemented in practice. Medicines play an increasingly important role in all aspects of patient care, particularly in hospital. As these medicines become more complex and patients present more difficult therapeutic challenges, the involvement of the hospital pharmacist will be vital for effective strategic medicines management.

References

1. Audit Commission. *A Spoonful of Sugar – Medicines Management in NHS Hospitals*. London: Audit Commission, 2001.
2. National Statistics. *Prescriptions Dispensed in the Community, Statistics for 1990–2000: England. Statistics Bulletin*. London: Department of Health, 2001.
3. Ministry of Health Central Health Services Council, Standing Pharmaceutical Advisory Committee. *Report of the Sub-committee on Hospital Pharmaceutical Services*. London: HMSO, 1955.
4. Nuffield Commision. *Report of the Nuffield Pharmacy Inquiry Committee*. London: Nuffield Foundation, 1986.
5. Department of Health. *Health Services Management: The Way Forward for Hospital Pharmaceutical Services*. HC(88)54. London: Department of Health, 1988.
6. Department of Health. *Pharmacy in the Future*. London: Department of Health, 2000.
7. Department of Health. *The Performance Management of Medicines Management in NHS Hospitals*. London: Department of Health, 2001.
8. Personal Communication. Office of the Chief Pharmacist for England. London: Department of Health, 2001.
9. Fitzpatrick R W, Mucklow J C, Fillingham D. A comprehensive system for managing medicines in secondary care. *Pharm J* 2001; 266: 585–588.
10. Walker D, Jackson C. Prescribing information in secondary care – the value of a national database? *Pharm J* 2000; 264: 263–265.
11. Ford N G, Curtis C, Paul R. The use of electronic prescribing as part of a system to provide medicines management in secondary care. *Br J Hosp Care* 2000; 17: 26–28.
12. NHS Executive. *Information for Health. An Information Strategy for the Modern NHS 1998–2005*. London: NHSE, 1998.
13. Fitzpatrick R W. Is there a place for drug and therapeutics committees in the new NHS? *Eur Hosp Pharm* 1997; 3: 143–147.
14. House of Lords Science and Technology Committee. *Resistance to Antibiotics and Other Antimicrobial Agents*. London: Stationery Office, 1998.
15. Standing Medical Advisory Committee Sub-group on Antimicrobial Resistance. *The Path of Least Resistance*. London: Department of Health, 1998.

16. *Hospital Prescribing Information Project – Final Report.* Liverpool: National Prescribing Centre, 1999.
17. Thomson S M. The role of the medicines management pharmacist. *Hosp Pharm* 1999; 6: 237–240.
18. Stephens M. Economic analyses to assist drug entry decision making. *Pharm Manage* 2001; 17: 36–40.
19. Barber N. Improving quality of drug use through hospital directorates. *Quality Healthcare* 1993; 2: 3–4.
20. Ketly D, Godfrey B D. Pharmacy and clinical directorates at Leicester Royal Infirmary. *Pharm J* 1992; 248: 588–589.
21. Edwards L. The role of the directorate liaison technician. *Hosp Pharm* 2000; 8: 115–116.
22. West Mercia Guidelines Partnership. Developing evidence based guidelines for general adult medicine. Presented at *The NICE Clinical Excellence – Spreading Good Practice Conference*, Harrogate, 1999.
23. Lord Hunt. Report of speech at NICE annual conference, London. *Pharm J* 2001; 267: 807.

Further reading

Audit Commission. *A Spoonful of Sugar – Medicines Management in Hospitals.* London: Audit Commission, 2001.

Fitzpatrick R W, Mucklow J C, Fillingham D. A comprehensive system for managing medicines in secondary care. *Pharm J* 2001; 266: 585–588.

Stephens M J, Tomlin M E, Mitchell R D. Managing medicines: the optimising drug value project. *Hosp Pharm* 2000; 7: 256–259.

9

Managing risk

Mark Tomlin

This book deals with the various functions seen in hospital pharmacy services: for each of them quality assurance and issues of quality of service have arisen. This chapter takes a broader view of several aspects of risk and quality assurance as they impact on hospital pharmacy. It addresses two government initiatives – controls assurance and clinical governance – moving on to describe issues of health and safety and clinical risk.

Controls assurance

In 1992 the Cadbury Committee produced a report on corporate governance [1]. This dealt with company directors' behaviour and how they would ensure their systems of internal control were effective. Corporate governance had been a theme in the National Health Service (NHS) for some time, dealing with probity in the finances of the service. Control of financial risks was the first step in the controls assurance programme [2]. In November 1999 this was extended to non-financial risks in an attempt to implement holistic risk reduction to underpin the delivery of quality care to patients. Controls assurance includes a series of standards which hospitals should achieve. It pulls together existing laws and regulations on a variety of areas into one cohesive structure [3]. Non-compliance with laws and regulations would mean that a trust is exposed to an additional risk; achieving controls assurance would mean that the laws are followed so risks are minimised.

The controls assurance programme also provides a system that informs trust boards about significant risks within the organisation. At the time of writing there are 21 controls assurance standards, listed in Table 9.1.

Table 9.1 Controls assurance standards

1	Buildings, land, plant and non-medical equipment
2	Catering and food hygiene
3	Decontamination of medical devices
4	Emergency planning
5	Environmental management
6	Financial standard
7	Fire safety
8	Governance standard
9	Health and safety
10	Human resources
11	Infection control
12	Information management and technology
13	Managing of purchasing and supply
14	Medical equipment and devices
15	Medicines management
16	Professional and product liability
17	Records management
18	Risk management system
19	Security management
20	Transport
21	Waste management

Medicines management – controls assurance standard

For pharmacy, medicines management is the most important controls assurance standard. The term 'medicines management' has been used in various ways over recent years [4–6]. The Audit Commission's definition of medicines management was given in chapter 7, encompassing all aspects of medicine use in hospital. The first draft of the controls assurance medicines management standard dealt largely with storage and supply of prescription-only medicines and controlled drugs [7]. Most hospitals had already written these regulations into their drugs policy and formulary systems [8]. Thus the initial document was criticised for falling short of the expectation of a modern pharmacy service, for example the activities of clinical pharmacy appeared to be omitted. A revised second version, including issues relating to drug usage and clinical pharmacy, was produced in February 2000 [9]. The standard aimed to test whether 'the organisation handles medicines safely and securely, in accordance with legislative requirements and best practice'. Local assessment against the criteria of the standard was undertaken in NHS trusts. A self-assessed score could be derived using a weighting system across the 18 criteria. In October 2001 a further revision was undertaken, attempting to widen the scope of the document to primary care trusts [10]. The document is a useful reference source for key pharmacy documents, as well as an audit tool. Table 9.2 lists the criteria of the October 2001 version; a draft revision was made available in autumn 2002 and the criteria remained the same [11].

The standard reinforces the concept that prescriptions must be written clearly and that the medicines supply route is through the pharmacy, including for clinical trials. It also makes clear that there should be pharmaceutical input into trial protocol and supports pharmaceutical input to local research ethics committees. It emphasises the need for a system to report, record and review known dispensing errors. The standard requires documented risk assessments and that these are supported by continuous monitoring, review and action plans to improve matters. It states that indicators to show improvements in safe and secure handling of medicines should be developed and that the trust board reviews medicines management-related risks.

Trusts will aim for scores above 75%; scoring below 40–50% could indicate that significant risks are present. Chief pharmacists lead on these issues and will put together action plans to reduce the risks – though reducing risk requires multidisciplinary effort.

Table 9.2 Controls assurance criteria October 2001

Criteria	Definition
1	Board-level responsibility and accountability defined
2	Controls in place to ensure Duthie Report [11] followed
3	Medicines are stored in safe and secure manner
4	Prescription charges are collected appropriately
5	Unlicensed dispensing complies with EL(97)52
	Licensed activities covered by specials licence
6	Prescription, supply and administration follow the legislation
	The activities are undertaken by qualified, competent staff
7	Controlled drug legislation is followed
8	Medicines waste is disposed of appropriately
9	Clinical trials work is undertaken appropriately
10	Adverse incidents involving medicines are dealt with appropriately
11	Supervision of dispensing is compliant with legislation
12	Risk management processes are applied to medicines management
13	Continuing professional development is undertaken
14	Access to up-to-date legislation and guidance is available
15	Resources to support the standard are available
16	Key indicators are available
17	The board monitors performance
18	Independent assurance of compliance is sought

Quality in the NHS

In 1997 the Department of Health published *The New NHS: Modern, Dependable* [12]. Though dealing with a wide range of organisational issues, it reemphasised that the NHS was about quality of care, not just about cost. In 1998 *A First Class Service: Quality in the New NHS* was produced [13]. It described an NHS where national standards would be set; these would be implemented consistently at a local level and would be monitored throughout the system. The National Institute for Clinical Excellence (NICE), along with National Service Frameworks, set the standards. Clinical governance would ensure dependable delivery, with monitoring by the Commission for Health Improvement (CHI) and surveys of patients and users of the service.

National Institute for Clinical Excellence

The government set up NICE to ensure that interventions and guidelines shown to benefit patients would be widely and consistently implemented throughout the NHS. NICE undertakes the technical appraisal of clinical techniques, equipment and supplies (including pharmaceuticals) as well as compiling clinical guidelines. This approach should ensure the rapid adoption of the best techniques, devices and therapies. It should also allow equity of access for patients, thus eliminating 'postcode prescribing' [12, 14].

The Medicines Control Agency assesses absolute clinical effectiveness, where a randomised clinical trial compares the new treatment against placebo and medicines are licensed if they have an effect – assuming there are not disproportionate risks. For their 'technology appraisals' (including medicines) NICE assesses the relative clinical effectiveness, where a randomised controlled trial compares a new initiative against the current standard. Cost-effectiveness is explored, where there is an examination of what benefits are achieved for the resources used.

NICE produces one of four recommendations:

1. Unrestricted NHS use
2. Use restricted to certain categories or indications
3. Use restricted to further trials and evaluations
4. NHS use not recommended.

Once issued, there is a requirement for trusts to implement guidance within 3 months. NICE advice has meant a significant growth in spend on medicines. Trusts should use NICE guidance to implement best practice and should conduct audit to test compliance with the standards.

Pharmacy clearly has a big part to play in this – ensuring dissemination, implementation and audit of guidance on medicine use.

Clinical governance

A First Class Service introduced the term 'clinical governance' and this has formed the basis of a major programme for NHS hospitals [13]. It represents a huge opportunity for pharmacy that has a potential impact on all areas. Clinical governance was, perhaps, a response to high-profile cases giving concern to the public, including the Bristol inquiry into deaths of children following cardiac surgery [15]. A key tenet of the document *A First Class Service* [13] was that clinical governance ensures an environment 'in which excellence can flourish'. The document provided the framework through which the NHS would be responsible for improving the quality of services and ensuring high standards of care. Chief executives became accountable for quality, not just financial balance.

The document had a number of themes:

- clinical governance:
    - — evidence-based practice and improving clinical effectiveness
    - — risk management
    - — use of information
    - — user involvement and complaints
- professional self-regulation
- lifelong learning.

Evidence-based practice and improving clinical effectiveness

There are hundreds of medical journals and thousands of papers published each year. It is beyond the ability of individuals to read them all. Even if this were possible, it is likely that the few gems of good research evidence would be lost in the quantity of poor research.

This plethora of information means that changes in practice are neither uniformly nor rapidly implemented. Clinical benchmarking has been built into practice to encourage a common best practice across the country. Each trust may devise local guidelines, initially for the benefit of junior staff, to ensure consistent patient care. Such guidelines have evolved into national guidelines and this has been taken further by the formation of NICE and the construction of National Service Frameworks.

Audit of local practice against local standards, or national standards, is an important way to test the quality of care. The move away from domination by the medical profession is illustrated by the change from medical audit (uniprofessional) to clinical audit (multiprofessional).

Integrated-care pathways are seen as a positive step forward in clinical effectiveness but their application tends to be limited to techniques such as thrombolysis, fractured neck of femur or coronary artery bypass grafting. An agreed multiprofessional plan of care is developed, often with standardised paperwork, so that 'standard care' is given to all patients – though room is made for exceptions to the norm.

Risk management

A key element of clinical governance systems is reducing clinical risks. This aspect is discussed later in the chapter.

Use of information

Clinicians need up-to-date and accurate information on the work they undertake if they are to achieve high-quality care. Information to monitor how well they are doing, to permit audit and to learn lessons is a key part of clinical governance. Information on a trust's performance may help the public decide where they wish to receive treatment. Broader information should also be available, such as annual reports describing what a trust has achieved and the outcomes of its efforts.

Within-trust policies and procedures could rapidly achieve wide consultation in their drafting or when changes are made. Currently hospitals receive a new printed *British National Formulary* every 6 months. If this were put on the trust intranet, everyone would have access.

The electronic patient records project is a major initiative. The idea is to have universal, multiprofessional notes accessible from any point in the hospital or even from general practitioner surgeries. This is to avoid current inefficiencies in lost notes, or notes in clinic when the patient is on the ward, or when two professionals need them at the same time. The infrastructure costs are huge and the changes in culture are only just beginning.

Internet access has already allowed professionals to read the latest specific product summary or data sheet from the Association of the British Pharmaceutical Industry website.

Complaints and user involvement

Complaints about the NHS should be seen as an opportunity to improve and change the service provided. Trusts are required to provide information to users of their service on how to complain, and to give timely responses when complaints arrive.

Patients and public representatives should be involved in the assessment of the quality of services. Patients' views should also be obtained when deciding whether to introduce new services or improve existing ones. Patients will comment on the total patient journey, not just clinical outcomes. If lessons are learnt this should increase client satisfaction and reduce complaints. Public consultation should ensure that services are user-friendly and meet the needs of all patients.

Lifelong learning

To complement clinical governance, *A First Class Service* [13] identified the need for lifelong learning. Continuing professional development was to be a key part of the NHS culture (including consultants). The aim is to ensure that staff have the knowledge and skills they need for the service. Chapter 13 deals with education and training issues within the pharmacy.

Professional self-regulation

A First Class Service [13] noted that professional self-regulation gives health professionals the ability to set their own standards of professional practice, conduct and discipline. Such freedom comes with duty – open accountability, building on the public's expectations and consistent application. Professionals should share their expert knowledge and experience of what works best and how to handle difficult situations. Professions should allow peer review and encourage clinical supervision and audit of practice. If professions did this they could safeguard the interests of the public and continue to regulate themselves, though with greater lay input to their governing bodies.

Pharmacy's role

Pharmacy departments need to implement systems to ensure that clinical governance is in place. There are also some important roles for pharmacy to play in the clinical governance programme outside pharmacy. Pharmacists can support the clinical effectiveness agenda on medicines and medicines use. Identifying, reporting, analysing adverse events and assisting change based on lessons learnt is another important role. Contributing to the education and development of others is another.

Commission for Health Improvement

CHI was established in 1999 to inspect the quality of services provided by the NHS. It is expected that all trusts will be visited every 4 years. Where trusts are failing the standards expected by CHI, new management will be imposed. CHI will test local clinical governance arrangements and the implementation of national guidance. CHI will work towards a common standard across the country.

Trusts that rank highly against CHI standards will be given greater freedom to allocate resources to their own priority projects. Middle-ranking trusts will have to seek approval for their own projects. The lowest-ranking trusts will not be allowed their own priorities. Revised arrangements are being developed at the time of writing to bring together several of the monitoring bodies, simplifying arrangements for inspection.

Risk management

Controls assurance standards have been discussed above; they seek to address risk issues in NHS hospitals. The remainder of this chapter will examine broader risk issues, beginning with health and safety matters, hazardous substances and moving on to clinical risk.

Health and safety

Health and safety deals with systems of work and the working environment. There is a need to question the suitability of facilities and equipment for the work undertaken as well as the adequacy of staff training [16–18]. Employers are responsible for providing a safe and healthy environment for staff. This is a legal responsibility under the Health and Safety at Work Act. Employees also have responsibilities – to ensure they use safety equipment, follow procedures and so on.

Areas of significant concern in hospitals include risk of fire, manual handling procedures, use of visual display units (VDUs), workplace stress, ionising radiation exposure and infection control.

Fire procedures and annual training help avoid injuries and death should a fire occur – these are in addition to good building design and alarm systems.

Sick leave may follow injury due to poor manual handling. A significant number of nurses have retired through ill health following a back injury caused by lifting patients inappropriately. Hospitals address this by extensive moving and handling training with regular refresher sessions [19]. Appropriate systems are needed for moving goods in pharmacy, using the right equipment and supported with good training.

VDU use must be monitored, with good workstation design and staff being offered appropriate eye tests [20].

Radiation protection and its specialist regulations should be studied if undertaking work with radiopharmaceuticals. Appropriate exposure monitoring must be undertaken. On the wards care must be taken in the use of X-rays as staff can receive significant cumulative dosing during their careers.

Violence to staff is an increasing problem in Accident and Emergency (A&E). Sick patients are frightened and confused and may be irrational, lashing out at those who are there to help them. A significant number of A&E attendees are under the influence of drugs and alcohol. Patients may be frustrated by treatment delay. Policies are being developed that support removal of those behaving unreasonably, unless their behaviour is a direct result of their illness.

Staff are provided with immunisation against hepatitis C and flu as their work exposes them to increased risk. Hospitals my grind to a halt in a flu epidemic if significant numbers of nurses are off sick. If insufficient nurses remain to care for the sick, this represents a risk which can only be managed by closing beds.

A no-smoking policy forms part of health and safety, in that it protects staff, reduces the length of time off sick and decreases future NHS workload. Patients wanting to smoke may be tempted to smoke in bed, with the attendant fire risk. It is not unknown for patients on oxygen therapy to be abusive to staff who refuse to let them have cigarettes.

In all aspects of health and safety the aim will be to remove the risks, and where this is not possible, to provide systems and training to minimise the consequences [21, 22].

The Control of Substances Hazardous to Health (COSHH)

The COSHH regulations require employers to evaluate and control the risks to health for all employees from exposure to hazardous substances [23]. This includes microbiological agents, dust in substantial quantities and all chemicals hazardous to health except lead and asbestos that are controlled by other regulations, as are radioactive materials.

Assessments are made and data sheets produced for the substances with an accompanying safety sheet. The data sheet covers the material, composition, usage, physical data, fire hazard and housekeeping issues.

The safety sheet covers health hazards, spillage, first aid and storage and handling.

Cytotoxics come under the regulations, as do all chemicals issued by pharmacy, from inhalation gases to disinfectants and poisons [24]. For example, gluteraldehyde has been widely used to disinfect endoscopy tubes, but is hazardous to staff by contact and inhalation. Safe ventilation systems are required and gluteraldehyde must be rinsed from instruments before insertion into the next patient. Pharmacy deals with strong acids, pharmacologically active compounds (e.g. testosterone cream), explosives such as hydrogen peroxide and inflammables such as alcoholic solutions. Safe systems are needed to handle these and staff need to understand the potential problems.

Clinical risk

Airlines have monitored risk closely over the years because of the potential for significant loss of life, negative publicity and financial loss. Safety checks and safe systems are built into everyday practice. The perception of risk can be perverse: airlines are seen as risky because one adverse event costs many lives, whereas for car travel, events are frequent but the loss at each event is small.

Investment in safety in airlines is expected to cost money and this is seen as a good thing. In health care safety is taken for granted and so is associated with minimal resources. However over recent years managing risks has risen on the agenda, perhaps in part due to the rise in litigation over negligence claims [25].

Clinical risks, like all others, can be viewed as having a 'likelihood' and a 'consequence'. The likelihood can be described as the chance, or probability, that an event can occur. The consequences define the seriousness of the risk – whether harm or even death can result. Risks which are very likely to occur and have severe consequences merit more attention than risks which are not likely to occur and which have trivial consequences.

Risk-free medicines

The general public expects medicines to be risk-free. Pharmacists do not suffer from this delusion and they spend their time minimising the risks of drugs [26, 27]. All drugs carry the risk of an adverse event [28, 29]. New products carry an additional risk because their full effects are unknown. There are also older products where the risks are well known but remain a significant cause for concern – potassium chloride injection is an example [30, 31].

Whilst the manufacture and distribution chain is well controlled, the usage of medicines is not. Putting this right is the *raison d'être* of clinical pharmacy [27, 32].

After diagnosis the doctor chooses a mode of treatment (surgical, pharmaceutical or radiological). If a medicinal product is required, the therapeutic group is chosen and then the individual agent. There are risks with the choice of therapeutic group as well as selection of agent within that group. Pharmacists, as experts in medicinal products, can reduce the risks of an adverse outcome or event by early communication with the prescriber.

Adverse drug reaction (ADR) reporting

The development of ADR reporting is illustrative of the evolution of risk management. In the early days reporting of ADRs would increase the knowledge base about the frequency and harm arising from medicines. Drugs with many ADRs would be excluded from formularies if their benefits did not justify the risks. Also, certain drugs could be avoided in given clinical circumstances where harm was likely [29]. There may have been reluctance to complete the 'Yellow Cards' partly due to a fear that blame would be apportioned. Refreshingly, all pharmacists can now complete the reports, and numbers of reports by pharmacists have increased [33, 34]. Pharmacists have an ability to evaluate harm and risk equal to that of the doctor [35, 36].

History of risk

Patient confidentiality has been a major principle of the medical profession and the health care service as a whole. Confidentiality of medical records is important, but this has built the mystique of medical practice and excluded clinical decisions and health care actions from any inspection or audit. This may have limited the opportunity to learn from adverse events.

An Organisation with a Memory made some of these previous principles explicit [37]. It also tried to generate an open culture where patient confidentiality was maintained, but poor clinical practice revealed.

Pharmacists have for many years recorded their activities on the wards. Interventions were documented to show workload and demonstrate the improvement in health care practice that the pharmacist could deliver. Recording pharmacists' interventions had another beneficial effect. It informed all pharmacists in a department what they were each doing, that is, sharing good practice. Discussion of interventions showed how they were performed, who had the knowledge and who could apply it. It also showed how good pharmacists were at communicating this knowledge and persuading medical staff to change their prescribing or nurses how to improve the administration of medicines. When collated and fed back to the pharmacy department, it raised the general awareness about which were the hazardous medicines, where clinical practice was prone to error and what incremental changes could be made to correct adverse events that had occurred, reducing or preventing the risks. Awareness of risk is the first step in reducing adverse consequences.

Adverse event reporting

In addition to adverse reaction reporting and pharmacist intervention monitoring, trusts have developed adverse event and near-miss reporting systems – sometimes called critical incident reports (CIRs). CIRs should be collated and shared with the health professionals involved so they can consider safety action plans. Central analysis by experts (including a pharmacist where medicines are involved) is important to test for generic errors such as a lack of skills for drug calculations or how to give injectables such as epidurals or intrathecals.

When a number of CIRs have been collected some common themes emerge. This may help in the initial sorting of the reports. However the real aim is to look for the factors which influenced or caused the events to occur in the first place. This is called root cause analysis.

Root cause analysis can best be achieved by a round-table discussion of all the health care professionals involved. The pharmacist is key to this discussion when medicines are involved and important even in non-pharmaceutical adverse events. This is because of the extensive training of pharmacists in the dispensing process. Understanding the product and the process is crucial to preventing errors creeping in. Familiarity with the breakpoints in this process means that pharmacists are good at process analysis, looking for efficiencies and areas of weakness. Pharmacists also have skills in process monitoring and reasons for deviation. On the wards clinical pharmacists, by intervening in the prescribing and administration of medicines, learn the weak points.

Common errors should persuade the pharmacist to rewrite the process so that it is safer or more efficient.

It important not to make assumptions or focus on a simple cause. Most events require more than one defect for an adverse event to occur. Barriers are built into best practice to prevent a hazard reaching the patient. However each barrier has holes, like a slice of Swiss cheese. Hazards get through when all the holes line up. It is important to accept that humans make errors so systems should be built to incorporate checks or make errors less likely.

It is increasingly apparent that pharmacists need to contribute to medical training. For many years now, junior doctors have appreciated the helpful words of the pharmacists. Now these same doctors are consultants they are encouraging input from pharmacists into clinical practice and medical undergraduate training.

Electronic prescribing systems are heralded as the solution to many prescribing errors [27]. Whilst they eliminate the trivial, it is important to be alert to the potential for creating new problems and concealing more complex ones.

Risk action

Having collected all this data, analysed it and discovered the root causes, what does one do about it? Many CIRs reveal a failure to follow the correct procedure. This has many root causes: lack of awareness that a procedure existed; lack of knowledge about the content of the procedure; lack of skill in executing the procedure; forgetting what to do. We can learn:

- It is important to publicise new or changed procedures through a news sheet or managerial briefing. Distribution on the hospital intranet enables staff to look for procedures even if they were previously unaware of their existence.
- Content of procedure has to be part of basic training and continuing education. Competency to practise should be based on the knowledge of the procedure or where to find the data. This raises the question of initial approval as well as continuous assessment.
- Skills training is already happening in the nursing profession and pharmacy may need to catch up here. One feels that community pharmacists undertaking prescribing analyses and cost (PACT) data analysis could learn from hospital formulary experiences. Assessment and audit of prescribing are integrated into clinical pharmacy but how well do we audit our own practice?
- The human memory is an elusive beast. Sometimes routines can be followed by reinforcement; sometimes they vanish without the awareness that they ever

existed. Repetitive process bores the brain yet this is fundamental to memory enhancement.

- Hospital management can help in initiating new policies and procedures that ensure that staff know what is expected of them. It is crucial that this is presented as adult learning and not patronising. The end is a common goal of improving patient care.

If procedures are written, staff are trained in them and the procedures are executed with skill then litigation can be avoided. So critical incident reporting can help to set standards and create awareness that a procedure needs auditing. It facilitates useful research and supports training. It aids re-engineering and improves patient care. The only catch is the resources required to undertake it and pay for the implementation of any action plans.

The clinical negligence scheme for trusts

To deal with litigation the NHS established the clinical negligence scheme for trusts (CNST). This provides different levels of insurance cover for protection against negligence claims. The level of compliance with a series of standards determines the size of the premium. Higher levels of risk management imply lower insurance premiums.

Conclusion

Developing a 'modern and dependable' NHS requires the consistent delivery of high-quality care. Controls assurance and clinical governance should both assist to build quality into the NHS. There is a declared intent to reduce the number of adverse events due to medicines; introducing reporting systems and gaining support for their use may result in increasing report numbers. However, if lessons are learned and actions taken, the 'true number' of events may begin to fall. Pharmacy has a key role in achieving this goal.

References

1. Cadbury Committee. *The Financial Aspects of Corporate Governance.* London: Burgess Science Press, 1992.
2. Department of Health. *Risk Management and Organisational Control Standards.* HSC 1999/123. London: Department of Health, 1999.
3. Department of Health. *Guidelines for Implementing Controls Assurance in the NHS.* London: Department of Health, 1999.

4. Tomlin M. Value analysis of hospital pharmaceutical services – pharmacy: expensive or valued? *Pharm Manage* 1997; 14: 2–4.
5. Stephens M, Tomlin M, Mitchell R. Managing medicines – Southampton's optimising drug value project. *Hosp Pharm* 2000; 7: 256–259.
6. Tweedie A, Jones I. What is medicines management? *Pharm J* 2001; 266: 248.
7. NHS Executive. *Medicines Management Controls Assurance Standards*, revision 01. London: NHS Executive, 1999.
8. Controls assurance: managing risk. *Pharm J* 2000; 265: 730.
9. Department of Health. *Medicines Management (Safe and Secure Handling)*. London: Department of Health, 2000.
10. Department of Health. *Medicines Management (Safe and Secure Handling)*, revised. London: Department of Health, 2001.
11. Department of Health. *Medicines Management (Safe and Secure Handling)*, revised. London: Department of Health, 2002.
12. Department of Health. *The New NHS: Modern, Dependable*. London: Department of Health, 1997.
13. Department of Health. *A First Class Service*. London: Department of Health, 1998.
14. NICE launched by Health Secretary. *Pharm J* 1999; 262: 490.
15. Bristol Royal Infirmary. *Learning from Bristol: the Report of the Public Inquiry into Children's Heart Surgery at the Bristol Royal Infirmary 1984–1995*. Command Paper CM5207. London: The Stationery Office, 2001.
16. HSE. *Health and Safety at Work Act Regulations*. London: HMSO, 1974.
17. HSE. *The Management of Health and Safety at Work Regulations*. London: HMSO, 1992.
18. HSE. *Workplace Health, Safety and Welfare*. London: HMSO, 1992.
19. HSE. *Manual Handling*. London: HMSO, 1992.
20. HSE. *Display Screen Equipment at Work*. London: HMSO, 1992.
21. HSE. *Work Equipment*. London: HMSO, 1992.
22. HSE. *Personal Protective Equipment at Work*. London: HMSO, 1992.
23. Department of Health. *Control of Substances Hazardous to Health* (COSHH). London: Department of Health, 1998.
24. Risk management in oncology. *Pharm J* 2000; 265: 732.
25. NPSA. *Doing Less Harm*. London: Department of Health, 2001.
26. Department of Health. *Pharmacy in the Future*. London: Department of Health, 2000.
27. Audit Commission. *A Spoonful of Sugar – Medicines Management in NHS Hospitals*. London: Audit Commission, 2001.
28. Cavell G. Medication errors are causing 'one or two' deaths every day. *Pharm J* 1995; 254: 716.
29. US data suggest adverse drug reactions could be a leading cause of death. *Pharm J* 1998; 260: 582.
30. Cousins D. KCl infusions also need care. *Hosp Pharm Pract* 1998; 8: 494.
31. Cousins D. Beware dosing errors with low molecular weight heparin. *Hosp Pharm Pract* 2000; 10: 260.
32. Tomlin M. Medication risk management – the pharmacist's role. *Hosp Pharm* 1999; 6: 314.

33. 'Yellow card' reporting now allowed for all community pharmacists. *Pharm J* 1999; 263: 776.
34. Davis S, Coulson R. Community pharmacist reporting of suspected ADRs: (1) The first year of the yellow card demonstration scheme. *Pharm J* 1999; 263: 278–791.
35. Martin R M, Mann R D, Hands D E *et al*. Design of a pilot prospective cohort study of adverse events monitoring by hospital pharmacists. *Int J Pharm Med* 1999; 13: 11–16.
36. Emerson A, Martin R, Tomlin M, Mann R. Prospective cohort study of adverse events monitoring by hospital pharmacists. *Pharmacoepidemiol Drug Safety* 2001; 10: 95–103.
37. Department of Health. *An Organisation with a Memory*. London: Department of Health, 2000.

Further reading

Audit Commission. *A Spoonful of Sugar – Medicines Management in NHS Hospitals*. London: Audit Commission, 2001.

Cousins D H. Why we must now act in theatre. *Hosp Pharm Pract* 1998; 8: 64–66.

Cousins D H. Communication is key to safety. *Hosp Pharm Pract* 1998; 8: 120–121.

Cousins D H, Upton D R. Errors in ICU must be stopped. *Hosp Pharm Pract* 1998; 8: 161–162.

Cousins D H, Upton D R. Improve PILs to avoid confusion. *Hosp Pharm Pract* 1998; 8: 294.

Daly M J, Marshall I W. Risk management in hospital pharmacy. *Pharm Manage* 1996; 12: 44–47.

Department of Health. *A First Class Service*. London: Department of Health, 1998. www.doh.gov.uk/riskman.htm (accessed 10 November 2002).

Pruce D, Remington H. Clinical governance for pharmacists in the managed services. *Hosp Pharm* 2001; 8: 198–199.

10

Community services pharmacy

Beth Taylor and Elaine Bartlett

Community health services (CHS) have often been viewed by hospital staff as a separate, and sometimes distant, part of the managed health service. It is true that CHS only became part of the National Health Service (NHS) in 1974, being managed by local authorities prior to this date. These diverse and locally variable services, often led by nurses or therapists, are provided from clinics, health centres and in people's homes. They are an important element in the health care of many older or disabled people, and of families with young children. This chapter describes CHS, how they link to social care and the support that is provided by pharmacists specialising in this area of practice (often known as community services pharmacists or CSPs).

History

In 1974, hospital pharmacy was undergoing a period of rapid development and many departments did not initially respond to the needs of these less familiar services, which had suddenly appeared within the portfolio of district pharmaceutical officers. Gradually, awareness developed and in the late 1970s, a few specific pharmacist appointments were made to cater for the needs of CHS staff. Initially, this activity focused on delivering traditional pharmaceutical supply services but, as most CHS staff had not previously had access to professional advice, there were many challenges. For instance, local enuresis clinics at this time would commonly order bulk supplies of drugs such as imipramine, and hand them out to parents in brown envelopes with the dose and child's name written on the front. Childhood vaccines could be stored in bulk in an office fridge, and then routinely sent to general practitioners (GPs) in the general post. Early CSPs aimed for CHS staff to receive the same level of pharmaceutical support that their colleagues working in hospitals had enjoyed for some years.

By 1986, numbers of CSPs had grown and a national specialist group was formed, with up to 300 members. The Community Services Pharmacists Group (now known as the Primary and Community Pharmacy Network) was established to provide peer support, networking and education opportunities to those working in this field. Spread of CSP posts across the country, and the seniority of such posts, has always been variable and often reflects the development of the CHS services in each area. A high proportion of posts are part-time, or sometimes linked to other duties within hospital pharmacy.

In the early 1990s, the creation of NHS trusts began to change the landscape. Instead of sitting within the overall umbrella of a district health authority, CHS services could be provided from one of three types of trusts. Many linked with mental health services, some remained as integrated, district-wide trusts and a few large urban areas had a big enough critical mass of services to form a separate community NHS trust. During this period, the strategy of a 'primary care-led NHS' led to a period of rapid development of many CHS. These organisational structures continued through the 1990s until the creation of primary care trusts (PCTs) from April 2000 onwards. In this latest restructuring, at long last community health and primary care staff find themselves working directly alongside each other within the same NHS organisation (see chapter 1 for details of NHS structures).

Key roles which have developed to support staff within CHS are supply, advice, information, education and training, monitoring safe practices with medicines and reducing medication-related risks.

The pharmacy services to community trusts providing CHS have historically been provided from a wide variety of sources, ranging from a directly employed team of pharmacists, technicians and support staff down to part of a single pharmacist's time provided from an acute trust. Pharmaceutical support has varied from a mainly supply-based service to well-developed clinical services with appropriate supply and dispensing arrangements for bedded services. Table 10.1 gives the range of services typically provided.

PCTs have the function of:

- improving the health of the community
- developing primary health services and CHS
- commissioning secondary care services.

They will need to develop and implement high-quality effective services, which must include the cost-effective and appropriate management of medicines.

Table 10.1 An example of the range of community health services provided in an urban area

Core services usually aligned to GP practices	Services usually provided on a wider or borough basis	Specialist services which are provided across a larger population
Health visiting	Teams caring for those with a physical disability	Developments such as walk-in centres
District nursing	Consultant community paediatricians	Specialist child health services
Chiropody (routine)	Immunisation and vaccination	Homeless and refugee team
Physiotherapy (routine)	Specialist health visiting	Home enteral nutrition team
	Continuing care of the elderly, including community hospitals	Home loans
	Specialist community teams, e.g. for learning disability	Rehabilitation services
	Palliative care	GP wards
	Community HIV/AIDs services	Tissue-viability nurse
	Family planning, including specialist clinics	Interpreting service
	Foot health services	Continence service
	Child protection	Diabetes resource team
		Podiatry
	Speech and language therapy	In-house pharmacy service
	School health	Infection control

GP, general practitioner; HIV, human immunodeficiency virus; AIDS, acquired immuno-deficiency syndrome.

It may well be the case that hospital pharmacists with their particular clinical expertise will increase and expand their relationship with PCTs to improve dialogue between primary, secondary and tertiary care. We already know that involvement in processes such as discharge planning between hospital, community and practice pharmacists at the interface has improved patient care and these links need to be extended and formalised. PCTs may still wish to purchase their pharmacy services from an acute hospital trust but will be much more focused in their requirements in the future.

Just as in community health trusts, PCTs still need to have appropriate structures in place to conform to all the standards surrounding medicines management, clinical governance and controls assurance (see chapter 9). Prescribing will have to be managed across primary and secondary care boundaries; management is about not just controlling costs but promoting cost-effective prescribing that improves the health of the population. It is likely that individual PCTs will develop their own, and sometimes very different, models and strategies and hospital pharmacy managers and staff will need to respond to these demands.

What are community health services?

The structure of the previous community health trusts differed across the country, as some also included learning disabilities, mental health and regional rehabilitation services. With the formation of PCTs, all CHS have migrated to new organisations.

It is important that hospital pharmacists and pharmacy managers understand the range of the clinical input and pharmaceutical services that will need to be provided to CHS within PCTs. Experience of the support which has already been provided to CHS provides a good basis on which to move forward to build future services. Some key roles have developed for pharmacists providing support to CHS.

Advice

PCTs will need to ensure that all CHS staff have access to appropriate professional pharmaceutical support. This must include the development and endorsement of appropriate medication policies such as:

- safe and secure handling and storage of medicines in all areas of use
- handling and use of cytotoxics
- treatment of anaphylactic shock
- safe disposal of unwanted medicines
- use of pharmaceutical samples
- disinfection
- handling, use and transport of vaccines
- head lice infection
- adverse reaction reporting

- mercury spillage
- hazard recall
- Control of Substances Hazardous to Health (COSHH).

Developments in prescribing and the supply and administration of medicines

Patient group directions (previously known as group protocols)

The increasing use of patient group directions (PGDs) for the administration and/or supply of appropriate prescription-only medicines is evident within CHS, for example in family planning, or walk-in centres. As it is a legal requirement that a pharmacist has involvement in writing and endorsing the use of such PGDs, CSPs have developed expertise in both writing and working with PGDs and there is a website where model PGDs have been posted [1, 2]. Table 10.2 gives some examples of PGDs used in community services.

Knowledge of the environment in which community health staff operate, for instance the way in which school vaccination sessions are organised, is essential in order to make PGDs workable and appropriate. They must be individually tailored to match the health professionals concerned and their working practices.

Pharmacists are also required to utilise their knowledge and expertise in legal issues surrounding medicines, and apply this to address the complex circumstances that community-based health staff often encounter.

Nurse prescribing

The introduction of nurse prescribing has been phased in gradually, starting in 1994, when the first demonstration sites involving health visitors and district nurses were established. This first phase, whereby

Table 10.2 Examples of patient group directions (PGDs) in use within community health services

Service	*PGD*
Family planning	Supply and administration of oral contraceptives
District nursing	Administration of flu vaccine
Health visitors	Administration of childhood immunisations
School nurses	Administration of childhood vaccines given at school

23 000 nurses in the UK with a health visitor or district nurse specialist qualification were trained and accredited to prescribe from the Nurse Prescribers' Formulary, was completed in March 2001. In January 2002, the second phase began to be rolled out, and an extended formulary for about 10 000 new nurse prescribers has been agreed. The two formularies are to be found in the back of the *British National Formulary* [3]. In contrast to the first phase, nurses are selected for training based primarily on the benefits to patients that this development might bring, and it is aimed primarily at minor ailments, minor injury, palliative care and health promotion services.

The NHS Plan signalled the introduction of supplementary prescribing [4]. A consultation on its introduction was undertaken in 2002 [5]. Nurse training for supplementary prescribing started in 2003 with pharmacist training beginning later that year. The proposed definition of supplementary prescribing is: a voluntary partnership between the responsible independent prescriber and a supplementary prescriber to implement an agreed patient-specific clinical management plan with the patient's agreement, particularly but not only in relation to prescribing for a specific non-acute medical condition or health need affecting the patient. It is anticipated that this will be of great benefit within the management of chronic illnesses such as diabetes and asthma, and may interest many more nurses than the relatively small numbers who might practise as independent prescribers.

Pharmacists have a critically important role in supporting this development, initially for nurse prescribers but in time this will extend to other professional groups such as therapists. To date they have contributed to university teaching courses, ongoing support, and monitoring of electronic prescribing analyses and cost (ePACT) data for nurse prescribers. As this develops, they will be required to ensure that consistent and safe prescribing practices are maintained across a more diverse group of practitioners.

Supply

The supply of basic medicines to staff in CHS has usually been provided by an acute trust under a service-level agreement. There may well be proposals by PCTs in the future to purchase and supply medicines in an innovative way. Such proposals will need careful professional and legal scrutiny to ensure that patients receive the most effective treatments available. The viability of other services such as community pharmacy must be carefully considered. Although appropriate and cost-effective use of pharmaceuticals must be monitored by a pharmacist, the supply function may be carried out by competent pharmacy technicians and assistant technical officers (ATOs). There should be written policies which comply with the Duthie Report [6] guidelines for safe and secure handling of medicines and the NHS Executive Controls Assurance Standards on Medicines Management [7]. Satisfactory procedures for ordering, supply and safe delivery of pharmaceuticals to community premises must be in place. Stock levels agreed between health professionals and the pharmacist must be available as a basis for ordering and stock control in every clinic. Safe and secure storage must be provided in community premises.

Vaccines

Vaccine supplies for GPs have historically often been provided by acute trusts but are now generally provided by a distribution company (Farillon) to GP practices. The Department of Health (DoH) has set up a contract with Farillon to provide a direct delivery service using refrigerated lorries. However, vaccines for the school nursing service, which provides immunisations within schools, according to the current DoH vaccination schedules, need to be ordered, stored and delivered to school nurses appropriately, maintaining an adequate cold chain and proper documentation and an audit trail at every stage. It is essential that the cold chain is maintained up to the point of delivery of the vaccine to the child in school. Advice on appropriate and verified cool boxes with monitoring of temperatures reached is also an essential part of the pharmacist's involvement.

Family planning

Family planning clinics provide free birth control advice and contraceptives to any person needing advice. The reduction of unwanted pregnancies is an important part of the government's sexual health strategy and the provision of oral contraceptives and other family planning items to clinics should be rationalised [8]. An accepted formulary allows the appropriate and cost-effective use of medicines within the service. The number of nurse-led clinics using PGDs is increasing and these need to have appropriate pharmacist input to ensure that both the PGDs and legal requirements, such as appropriate labelling of oral and emergency contraceptives, are being met.

Dentists

Dental clinics provide dental care for the community with particular emphasis on school children, antenatal and postnatal women, the physically handicapped, people with learning disabilities and domiciliary care for such patients unable to attend a clinic. Most individual patient treatment is provided on FP10 prescription but dentists obviously need local anaesthetics and other appropriate pharmaceuticals. General anaesthesia is now almost exclusively performed in a hospital setting but community dentists need to comply with current guidelines for dental emergencies such as anaphylactic shock and cardiac arrest. Provision of a supply service must always therefore be complemented by appropriate pharmaceutical advice.

Podiatrists

Podiatrists within the CHS are state-registered and provide services to the same group of patients as dentists together with the elderly. State-registered podiatrists who hold a certificate of competence in the use of medicines issued by or with the approval of the Podiatrists Board may sell or supply certain medicines in the course of their professional practice [9]. It is important to ensure that proper labelling requirements are being met. If they also hold a certificate of competence in the use of analgesics they may administer certain local anaesthetics parenterally. Podiatrists are also included in the list of health professionals who may be eligible to prescribe in the future. Many podiatrists also now provide services within GP practices. Again it is important that pharmacists providing a supply service to podiatrists satisfy themselves that appropriate guidelines and advice exist.

District nurses

District nurses are registered general nurses with a postregistration specialist qualification providing skilled nursing to patients within their own homes or in a GP surgery or clinic. All district nurses are now based within PCTs and may move between GP practices. District nurses are now eligible to become accredited nurse prescribers, prescribing from a limited list of medicines providing they have fulfilled the educational requirements. The majority of pharmaceutical items which they use should be obtained on FP10 or private prescription but sufficient stocks of dressings or non-prescription medicines may be supplied to enable them to initiate treatment.

Some nurses develop specialist expertise in defined areas such as stoma care, diabetes, paediatrics, continence and palliative care and need appropriate pharmaceutical advice rather than supplies.

Health visitors

Health visitors are registered general nurses with a postregistration qualification who are responsible for the health and development of the family, particularly relating to children under 5 and the elderly. The requirement for pharmaceutical supplies for health visitors is minimal. Health visitors provide advice on health promotion and preventive medicine and need pharmaceutical advice on topics such as drugs in breast milk, medicines in pregnancy, treatment of head lice infection, immunisation and medicines in children and the elderly. It is important that health visitors give current and appropriate advice on topics such as immunisation and head lice infection and there is an important role for pharmacists in training and providing information.

Information

The provision of information and advice on medicine-related issues to community health staff and, where appropriate, to the public is a key role for pharmacists working with CHS. There should be access to a medicines information department and clear lines of communication should be agreed so that urgent queries can be answered quickly. The same standards of logging and documenting queries and checking content are applied as exist in information departments in hospitals. Community services pharmacists also produce active information such as regular bulletins on appropriate topics and single-subject newsletters on specific issues. Although as yet few community nurses may be able to access the internet, some sites are being developed to meet their needs.

Education and training

It is often the role of pharmacists within community health to identify relevant training needs of health care staff in the community, who often work in isolation and find it difficult to maintain their professional development. With the introduction of nurse prescribing, this has become an even more vital role which needs to be supported by all pharmacists working in CHS, within primary care and community pharmacy. Competencies must be agreed and developed within the new organisations. Within community and primary care, multidisciplinary working is vital and the expertise of other disciplines must be included. Pharmacists themselves also need to maintain professional competency and it is here that membership of support groups and the networking opportunities they provide are so useful.

Monitoring safe practices with medicines

Knowledge of the working practices of community health staff is essential in formulating policies for safe use of medicines. Procedures and policies written for hospitals rarely translate satisfactorily into the community. For example, the intramuscular administration of a cytotoxic medicine by a district nurse to a patient at home produces different problems to administration on a ward. Policies need to reflect how good practice may be applied in the individual setting. Multidisciplinary working is a fact of life in the community and the pharmacist may be called upon to advise on and monitor many diverse issues around medicines. The introduction of clinical governance means that standards around the use of medicines must be continually monitored and improved.

Supporting the implementation of public health programmes

Public health issues dealing with the prevention of disease and the promotion of health are currently at the top of the government's agenda. The public health white paper *Saving Lives: Our Healthier Nation* looks at improving health across all sectors of the population [10]. Initiatives such as smoking cessation clinics, and the reduction of pregnancy in young people have been started both within CHS and in primary care, and the move of CHS into PCTs mean there is an opportunity to rationalise these with support from primary care pharmacists, community pharmacists and CSPs. Walk-in centres have sprung up in many cities and many of these are staffed by nurses employed by PCTs. Many CSPs are involved in the management of medicines within them. As these clinics are nurse-led, the writing and endorsement of PGDs are an important part of the pharmacist's role.

School nursing and school vaccination programmes

Within the CHS school nursing has perhaps changed rather less than other services. School nurses are responsible for the health of children in primary and secondary school both in providing medical checks at key stages of development and in implementing the school vaccination programme, which includes school-leaver boosters and the BCG programme. The schedule for vaccination of school children has changed over the years but the profile of school nurses was dramatically increased in 1994 by the introduction of a mass immunisation programme against measles and rubella. There was a fear at this time that there would be a measles epidemic unless rapid action was taken. The campaign was almost exclusively led by nurses and proved the value of the school vaccination programmes in reducing morbidity and mortality from infectious diseases. CSPs were extensively involved in facilitating all the pharmaceutical aspects of the measles/rubella programme and worked with the DoH and the nursing services to ensure its success.

In 1999, building on the effectiveness of the measles/rubella campaign, the DoH initiated a campaign of mass vaccination against meningitis C of children and young people between the ages of 5 and 18, together with students in further education. This too has produced a dramatic reduction in meningitis C, particularly in the 'at-risk' age groups. Pharmacists were involved in developing the programme and supporting school nurses in its implementation. Currently an accelerated BCG programme has been reintroduced after a shortage of vaccine.

Because it is likely that other mass immunisation campaigns for school children will be implemented in the future, it is important that pharmacists continue to be involved with the school vaccination programme within PCTs.

Residential and nursing home – inspection and training

Before 1984 and the introduction of the Registered Homes Act, the pharmaceutical inspection of nursing homes had been done on an ad hoc basis, usually by district pharmaceutical officers. As CSPs became more involved with inspection, a need was identified for standards around both medicine management in homes and the inspection process. This led the Community Services Pharmacists Group to write *Guidelines for Registration and Inspection of Private Nursing Homes* in England and Wales and also guidelines for private hospitals, which became the national standards [11]. The 1984 Act did not set national standards in law, but allowed health authorities, as the registering bodies, to interpret the Act locally. CSPs are involved in the registration and inspection process and also in training both staff in care homes and pharmacists in the inspection process.

The Care Standards Act 2000 has been introduced to modernise the current regulatory system for social services and nursing homes. Its aims are greater clarity, consistency and quality of national standards for providing care services. The management of medicines within care homes is obviously a key factor in the provision of quality care and CSPs with experience of regulation have been involved in producing standards in all the major areas of care. The National Care Standards Commission (NCSC) has been set up to regulate social services and private health care and was in full operation from 1 April 2002. Further changes in regulations are planned in order to bring together both health and social care regulatory organisations. It is a requirement that pharmacists must still be involved in the regulation and inspection process. Some are directly employed by the NCSC, but there will be a need for other pharmacists, perhaps on a sessional contract basis, to inspect and advise on medicines in care homes. These pharmacists may come from a variety of backgrounds, including acute and primary care, utilising the experience gained by CSPs. As the new standards are implemented, there will also be a need for pharmacists to be involved in training both care staff and other inspectors.

Supporting intermediate and continuing care services for the elderly

In some trusts, community-based services for older people are managed alongside CHS, and often CSPs are involved in providing a service to them. These services include both those falling under the definition of intermediate care (that is, rehabilitation programmes of not more than 6 weeks) and long-stay or continuing care. Examples of the former include some community hospitals, rehabilitation teams, step-down units and other nurse-led services. Continuing care may be provided from NHS-run nursing homes, community hospitals or other similar facilities. As part of the implementation of the National Service Framework (NSF) for older people, the number of intermediate care beds available is set to rise, and there is likely to be further investment by government in this type of care in order to reduce inappropriate use of hospital beds [12]. Patients receiving this care may need help with self-administration of their medication and accessible information and their carers may also need support. Pharmacists can also help achieve effective communication between GPs and services around medication, particularly for respite care.

Support for people with learning disabilities

Since the mid-1980s, almost all large institutions which provided care for people with learning disabilities have been closed and replaced by a range of locally based services, which aim to integrate them as far as possible within local communities. A large number of group homes, hostels and nursing homes are now in existence, and a multidisciplinary community learning disability team usually coordinates any specialist health care required. Pharmacists may contribute to this team, along with therapists, specialist nurses and consultants. In addition, they may work with organisations providing health and social care to ensure that there are safe systems for the management of medicines in these settings. Some community mental health services may be organised on a similar basis and so similar pharmacy support may be provided.

This type of activity often needs to work alongside the support provided by community pharmacists who are advising staff in registered care homes for people with learning disabilities or mental health problems. However, many small homes or hostels may not be registered and therefore it is important to ensure that this professional support is made available through another route.

Working with other agencies

Social services

Local authorities are responsible for commissioning the social care needed by their residents, particularly children and vulnerable groups such as older people. These needs include access to care homes, domiciliary care, meals on wheels, fostering services, adoption, social care assessments, and occupational therapy, amongst many others. Increasingly, local authorities are encouraged by successive governments to outsource these services from the private or voluntary sector, and this has led to an expansion of private home care agencies and similar provision.

Although very few health staff such as nurses will be employed, many social care workers are involved with medication in the course of their duties. In care homes, they routinely administer medication to their residents, as do domiciliary home care workers. Both groups need to access training, professional advice and medicines information from pharmacists. While community pharmacists will provide support to individual clients and carers, CSPs will commonly work with the employing organisations to support safe practices with medication, including local policies, training programmes and documentation.

New systems for assessing a person's health and social care needs are being introduced as part of the *National Service Framework for Older People* [12]. The ability to benefit from medication will be included in this assessment process. These systems should lead towards closer integration of care, and more effective, person-centred ways of delivering services.

Local education authorities

Together with other health professionals such as specialist school nurses and community paediatricians, CSPs work with education authorities to ensure that there are proper policies for the control and use of medicines within both mainstream and special schools. Teachers and other school staff have historically been resistant to keeping or administering medicines within schools and many teachers are still worried about administering drugs such as methylphenidate for the treatment of attention-deficit hyperactivity disorder. However, teaching unions and education authorities now accept and endorse properly agreed medicine policies. Staff are fully indemnified by the education authorities for their actions if they have participated in appropriate in-service training and this is an area where CSPs continue to play an active part. Pharmacists also provide advice on topics such as treatment of head lice across an education authority and work to support school nurses and health visitors.

Voluntary agencies

Many of the voluntary agencies, such as Help the Aged, Age Concern and Parkinson's Disease Society, have concerns around the proper use of medicines by their clients. Supporting their health professional colleagues, CSPs give talks to individual self-help groups such as stroke clubs and give advice to agencies in formulating information leaflets on the use of medicines. Pharmacist involvement is essential and with the move of CHS to primary care it should become possible for input to be provided by the most appropriate pharmacy service.

The future

CSPs have had to adapt the way they have supported CHS staff throughout this period of change. Despite the frequent restructuring, core services to patients must remain and services such as district nursing, health visiting and school nursing have perhaps changed less than their employing organisation. However, CSPs now have to consider how to respond to the new challenges presented within PCTs. These new organisations directly employ CHS staff and probably, over time, most CSPs, and the need for pharmacy support and input will increase rather than diminish. There will be enormous opportunities to integrate primary health services and CHS as well as including social care – particularly if care trusts develop. By 2005, we can envisage a future in which they are based in primary care, but working alongside prescribing support pharmacists, community pharmacists, nursing, therapy and medical colleagues to support the use of medicines. The old role definitions may slowly disappear as a breed of new 'primary care pharmacist', encompassing all the differing medicines management skills of predecessors, emerges.

References

1. NHS Executive. *Patient Group Directions*. HSC 2000/026. London: Department of Health, 2000.
2. www.groupprotocols.org.uk. NHS-approved website for patient group directions (accessed 10 November 2002).
3. Nurse Prescribers' Formulary. In: *British National Formulary*, 44th edn. London: BMA and RPSGB, 2002: 774–779.
4. Department of Health. *The NHS Plan*. London: The Stationery Office, 2000.
5. Medicines Control Agency. *Consultation on Supplementary Prescribing*. MLX 284. London: Medicines Control Agency, 2002.
6. Department of Health. *Guidelines for the Safe and Secure Handling of Medicines: A Report to the Secretary of State for Social Services – The Duthie Report*. London: Department of Health, 1988.
7. NHS Executive Controls Assurance Standard on Medicines Management. Revision 02 (October 2001) www.open.gov.uk/doh/riskman.htm (accessed 12 May 2002).
8. Department of Health. *The National Strategy for Sexual Health and HIV*. London: Department of Health, 2001.
9. The Royal Pharmaceutical Society of Great Britain. *Medicines, Ethics and Practice – A Guide for Pharmacists*, 26th edn. London: RPSGB, 2002.
10. Department of Health. *Saving Lives: Our Healthier Nation*. London: The Stationery Office, 1999.
11. *Guidelines for Registration and Inspection of Private Nursing Homes*. Primary and Community Care Pharmacy Network at www.pccpnetwork.org/publications.asp (accessed 13 November 2002).
12. Department of Health. *National Service Framework for Older People*. London: The Stationery Office, 2001.

Further reading

www.nmhct.nhs.uk/pharmacy/pcclg.htm – papers by the Pharmacy Community Care Liaison group including: pharmacy support for people with learning disabilities February 1999. Pharmaceutical support to PCTs June 2001. (accessed 13 November 2002).

www.druginfozone.org/community_health/index.html – this medicines information site has a section dedicated to community health-related information (accessed 13 November 2002).

www.pccpnetwork.org – this site is maintained by the national group representing community services pharmacists (accessed 13 November 2002).

www.rpsgb.org.uk/nhsplan/index.html – a site hosted by RPSGB, which aims to support pharmacists in responding to the NHS Plan and pharmacy strategy (accessed 13 November 2002).

11

Information technology

Keith Farrar and Ann Slee

The Audit Commission's review of medicines management in hospitals sets out a vision of the use of information technology (IT) in hospital pharmacy:

> New medication is agreed between members of the clinical team and ordered at the bedside through a radio computer link to an automated dispensary, where robotic systems pick the new medicines and dispatch them to the patient's ward via a pneumatic tube [1].

At the time of writing this vision is probably a long way off for many, but in a small number of hospitals it is very close to full implementation. This chapter will examine the developments in IT as they apply to hospital pharmacy practice. We will identify the main developments in IT in hospital pharmacy, including electronic data interchange (EDI) and its impact on pharmacy procurement, the use of stock control systems, electronic prescribing and medicines administration, electronic patient records (EPRs) and pharmacy care plans, medicines information systems and the use of automation.

History

Computerised stock control systems were introduced to pharmacy during the 1980s to provide machine-generated labels [2, 3]. Some of these systems also provided limited management information about what drugs had been used and by whom. Systems were further developed to provide automatic stock control, patient medication records and drug interaction warnings. Despite these advances, many systems are still not used to their full potential.

Information sources have been revolutionised by the advance of the worldwide web but the use of IT in medicines information had early beginnings, with access to microfiche databases, such as Iowa and

Pharmline, while online searching via third-party online services such as Datastar followed soon after.

Electronic prescribing and the EPR were introduced into a number of hospitals in the USA in the 1970s but were first introduced into the UK in the early 1990s. The publication of *Information to Health* in 1998 [4] set out an ambitious timetable for the introduction of the EPR, including electronic prescribing. More recent developments, heralded in *Pharmacy in the Future*, include the introduction of automation to the supply process [5].

Electronic data interchange

One of the biggest areas for miscommunication when ordering and receiving medicines comes in the transmission of the order to the supplier. Traditionally, orders from regular suppliers, such as wholesalers, relied on telephone conversations, sometimes supported by faxed copies of the orders but more routinely by a posted hard copy. One of the earliest developments was to use supplier-specific hardware that allowed the electronic transmission of orders, using product codes (for example, prosper), via a telephone link. Whilst these systems reduced miscommunicating orders to some extent, they were labour-intensive for both the purchaser and the supplier. The aim of EDI was to allow information to be transferred from the purchaser's computer system to that of the supplier without the need for this information to be rekeyed. Transferring the information back again in terms of an electronic invoice is a development that, sadly, is still in its infancy.

The barriers to seamless transfer of information for ordering and invoicing purposes are similar to those that prevent seamless electronic transfer of prescription information into dispensary systems, namely the development of a standard drug database. Had more effort been put into solving this problem during the early days of electronic purchasing it is likely that electronic transfer of prescribing/drug information would have been facilitated.

Despite more than a decade of development there remain some pharmaceutical suppliers that cannot trade using EDI, meaning that a wholly electronic model is still out of reach.

The ideal would be a stock control system that determines what needs to be ordered; this would then be reviewed by a decision support system which double-checks that the order is correct, and then the order would be placed electronically. The goods when received would be checked by bar code against the delivery note and original order, to minimise delivery errors. The electronic invoice would then be checked automatically against the recorded delivery information and, via a decision support price checking system, validated invoices would be paid electronically. Human intervention would only be required if there were any exceptions defined by the decision support that was in place.

Stock control systems

Perhaps the earliest IT to be introduced into pharmacy practice, stock control systems allowed the production of a clear printed label, often with some information support about interaction checking. Many systems produced limited management information allowing pharmacists to review the use of medicines – by speciality, for example. This drug use review was particularly helpful to the financial side of medicines management and it has been extensively used in the USA. There the use of systems for billing purposes has ensured good-quality data capture and reporting. The provision of drug expenditure information showing month-on-month comparisons and top 50 expenditure items on a trust or at speciality level is common practice. We underestimate the ease with which such information becomes available due to its routine collection during the supply and dispensing process. To collect such information manually would be an impossible task in most large hospitals.

The introduction of patient medication records, common in community pharmacies, has had limited application in hospital practice but has potential advantages in operational terms. It could be used to reduce unnecessary redispensing and facilitate the re-engineering of supply and also in tracking expenditure in high-spending specialities such as haematology, in the treatment of human immunodeficiency virus (HIV) or areas where billing may be required.

Sadly, systems are still not as developed or utilised as they might be. There is no standard for such systems to define the type of information required or ordering algorithms; drug files are maintained at each site, interfaces with third-party databases are in their infancy and there is no requirement for an up-to-date system to be in place.

Part of the standard specification should include the capacity to interface with other systems, particularly EPR systems but also EDI gateways and automatic picking systems. One of the barriers to this seamless electronic transfer of information is the lack of a common drug file. This issue now requires urgent central action. The Department of Health and the National Health Service (NHS) Information Authority are working to produce a common drug file via the UK Standard Clinical Products Reference Source Project (UKCPRS) project, which is due to complete its work by 2004 [6].

Electronic patient record

The advancement of computer systems in the USA has demonstrated the potential advantages of the introduction of EPRs, with many of the benefits related to the introduction of electronic prescribing systems. Whilst introduction of these systems into the UK is still very limited, the government's stated ambition is to have EPR systems including electronic prescribing systems in place in all acute hospitals by 2005. The recent report from the Treasury, the Wanless Report, further underlined the importance of investment in IT [7].

One of the major benefits to accrue from such systems arises from physician order entry which requires the doctor to input requests for new medicines, X-rays or other investigations into the system directly. This physician order entry has been a feature of most UK applications whereas the health system in the USA, delivered as it is by independent private physicians, does not lend itself to mandatory requirements for physician order entry. As a consequence, despite having advanced computer systems, many of the advantages of an electronic record are missed due to lack of physician involvement with the system.

The use of EPR systems has shown a number of benefits in terms of improving communication and reducing risks to patients. A patient safety internet site (the Leapfrog Group – www.leapfroggroup.org) has estimated that computerised physician order entry could lead to the avoidance of 522 000 serious medication errors each year in the USA. This has been demonstrated in terms of improved legibility and completeness of prescriptions and quite dramatic improvements in patient care, with reduction in risks associated with inappropriate dosing or drug choice [8, 9]. Advanced systems that include clinical decision support with dose and interaction checking or checks of the appropriateness of the prescription already exist, allowing review of the prescription at the point of decision-making [10–12]. These systems have also been shown to be beneficial in the management of formulary drug choice [13].

One of the most significant challenges for the introduction of IT is the cultural change required for the successful implementation of these systems [14]. There are a number of difficulties in getting buy-in from a range of different professional groups. This seems particularly true for electronic prescribing, which has proved the most difficult application to introduce to most computerised health systems. Successful implementation requires strong clinical champions, a commitment from the highest level in the organisation and a clear expression of the clinical benefits for patients to be gained from the introduction.

Prescribing is an activity that affects almost every patient admitted to hospital and requires the active participation of the majority of hospital staff. It is also an area that must be fail-safe and there is no leeway for mistakes to be made. It is an area that, to many, seems too complicated to implement and often most enthusiasm for implementation comes from pharmacy. There are real clinical benefits to accrue from the implementation of electronic prescribing and the government quite rightly included this in its information for health agenda: the growing awareness of the need to manage medication errors raised by *An Organisation With a Memory* may give further stimulus to the introduction of electronic prescribing [15].

One of the barriers to the roll-out of EPR is undoubtedly the perceived cost of introducing an integrated information system. Most hospitals have some degree of IT implementation at the department level with systems such as patient administration, outpatient scheduling and often lab ordering and results reporting available within outpatient departments or even at ward level. As a consequence the IT budget for most hospitals is probably sufficient to support the introduction of an integrated system if spread over the lifetime of the system. However the perceived procurement and implementation costs are still the biggest barrier to the implementation of government strategy in this area. An announcement of additional funding for IT should go a long way to alleviate these reservations [16]. In fact, there is growing evidence that the introduction of electronic systems would actually be resource-releasing, as has been the case in other industries [17].

For those who have introduced such systems, these have tended to be imported from the USA and have required quite extensive local work to anglicise the existing system. There is clearly a case to be made for a more centralised approach to the tailoring of existing systems for the UK market, as system development currently tends to be based in the country of origin (almost universally the USA). This is an issue, given the rapid changes in technology, if we are to try to optimise the benefits that could accrue from the introduction of such systems.

The features of an ideal system are that it should be fast, reliable, locally adaptable to meet user preferences, fast, easy to learn and intuitive in its use, fully integrated or allow easy interfacing with other systems (such as departmental systems or medical devices and automated systems), fast and allow easy access to patient data for audit purposes (as well as patient care). In case clarification is needed – it must be fast. The debate between fully integrated hospital information systems or interfaced 'best-of-breed' systems is fiercely contested amongst the varying proponents. Our own preference is for a fully integrated system that allows users to view relevant data from other applications such as pathology when prescribing medicines such as warfarin or insulin or drugs with a narrow therapeutic index. Whichever option you choose, it is imperative to be able to see the system in operation at a working site and not just accept the impressive demonstration that the vendors offer.

Automation

Pharmaceutical wholesalers have demonstrated the business case for the introduction of automated picking systems. The introduction of these into hospital practice has been delayed by the historical supply chain process that existed with medicines being dispensed for limited periods to supplement ward stock during inpatient care and then resupplied, normally for 1 week, on discharge. This process did not facilitate the use of patient packs and the use of bulk dispensing packs was normal. However *Pharmacy in the Future* [5], reinforced by the medicines management framework, has advocated the introduction of dispensing for discharge, requiring an original pack to be supplied as soon as possible after admission. This has opened the door for the introduction of automated picking systems into hospital practice, bringing with it the realisation that the UK medicines market is not as flexible as it needs to be.

Evaluation of automated systems has produced mixed results, with different types of systems being evaluated in different settings (automated bedside medication dispensing systems in American wards or robotic systems in UK pharmacies). This is hardly surprising. Findings from a UK-based study show that automation reduced dispensing errors by almost 50% and released 31% of dispensing technician time for other duties [18].

If we are to maximise the benefits of IT and automation we need there to be some changes in the supply of medicines and how these medicines are packaged. In the same way that the desire to minimise risk in the USA drove the introduction of unit packaged doses, we need to see the introduction of a range of pack sizes that facilitate the initiation of new treatment without leading to excessive waste from part-used packs. We also need the introduction of a standardised bar code on medication packs which is unique to that pack and contains information about the supplier, the approved name, form and strength of the product, the pack size and the batch number and expiry date of the contents. The introduction of such a code would facilitate the supply chain process, allowing accurate booking-in of medicines as well as automated dispensing [19]. It would also allow bar checking of drug administration – evidence from medication error studies indicates that a third of all errors occur at the administration process. Introduction of such a robust checking system would go a long way towards reducing clinical risks to patients.

Conclusion

IT offers significant advantages to both patient care and to pharmacy practice. Electronic prescribing systems, with integrated knowledge-based checks for dose and drug and other interactions, that interface directly with automated dispensing systems will allow pharmacy staff to spend their time where it's of most value – with the patient. The growing support for such systems suggests that these will indeed be introduced into clinical practice within the next 5–10 years. In its most recent report (*A Spoonful of Sugar*), the Audit Commission suggests that the introduction of automated dispensing systems would virtually eliminate the current shortfall in technician numbers [1]. However, implementation of IT requires a significant effort on behalf of organisations. The cultural change required to ensure effective implementation is a much greater challenge than finding the right technology and, without the support of staff, systems such as robotic dispensers are just expensive shelving.

References

1. Audit Commission. *A Spoonful of Sugar – Medicines Management in NHS Hospitals*. London: Audit Commission, 2001.
2. Hospital computer package from Pharmed. *Pharm J* 1980; 225: 329.
3. Hughes I R. Computer systems in pharmacy: II. *Br J Pharm Pract* 1982; 4: 15–24.
4. NHS Executive. *Information for Health. An Information Strategy for the Modern NHS 1998–2005*. London: NHS Executive, 1998.
5. Department of Health. *Pharmacy in the Future – Implementing the NHS Plan*. London: HMSO, 2000.
6. www.nhsia.nhs.uk/ukcprs/pages/default.asp (accessed 13 November 2002).
7. Wanless D. *Securing Our Future Health: Taking a Long-term View. Final Report*. London: HM Treasury, 2002.

8. Hughes D K, Farrar K T, Slee A L. The trials and tribulations of electronic prescribing. *Hosp Presc Eur* 2001; 1: 74–76.
9. Evans R S, Pestotnik S L, Classen D C *et al*. A computer-asisted management program for antibiotics and other antiinfective agents. *N Engl J Med* 1998; 338: 232–238.
10. Bates D W, Leape L L, Cullen D J *et al*. Effect of computerized physician order entry and a team intervention on prevention of serious medication errors. *JAMA* 1998; 280: 1311–1316.
11. Raschke R A, Gollihare B, Wunderlich T A *et al*. A computer alert system to prevent injury from adverse drug events. *JAMA* 1998; 280: 1317–1320.
12. Hunt D L, Haynes R B, Hanna S E, Smith K. Effects of computer-based clinical decision support systems on physician performance and patient outcomes: a systematic review. *JAMA* 1998; 280: 1339–1346.
13. Slee A, Farrar K. Formulary management – effective computer systems. *Pharm J* 1999; 262: 363–365.
14. Lively B T, Shrader K R. High tech and the human condition: impact on employees. *Am Pharm* 1986; 26: 24.
15. Department of Health. *An Organisation with a Memory*. London: Department of Health, 2000.
16. www.doh.gov.uk/ipu/whatnew/deliveringit/nhsitimpplan.pdf (accessed 13 November 2002).
17. Abu-Zayed L A, Farrar K, Mottram D R. Comparative evaluation of systems for drug supply to hospital wards in the United Kingdom. *J Soc Adm Pharm* 2001; 18: 136–142.
18. Slee A, Farrar K, Hughes D. Implementing an automated dispensing system. *Pharm J* 2002; 268: 437–438.
19. Chester M I, Zilz D A. Effects of bar coding on a pharmacy stock replenishment system. *Am J Hosp Pharm* 1989; 46: 1380–1385.

Further reading

NHS Executive. *Information for Health. An Information Strategy for the Modern NHS 1998–2005*. London: NHS Executive, 1998.
Slee A, Farrar K. Formulary management – effective computer systems. *Pharm J* 1999; 262: 363–365.
Slee A, Farrar K, Hughes D. Implementing an automated dispensing system. *Pharm J* 2002; 268: 437–438.

12

Research and development

Sarah Hiom

This chapter aims to explain key historical events in the National Health Service (NHS) which have influenced practitioner approach to research. It discusses how to start a research or development project, looking at literature searching, funding streams within the NHS, methodological design, ethical considerations and how to disseminate findings. Finally some thoughts on future developments are discussed.

Definitions

Pharmacy practice research (PPR)

PPR attempts to investigate the way in which pharmacy is practised, in order to support the objectives of the profession. It ensures that pharmacists' knowledge and skills are used to best effect in resolving relevant problems in the NHS and meeting the multidisciplinary health needs of the population [1].

Audit

Audit is a means of quality assurance where practice is monitored against set predetermined standards of care or practice. Audit demonstrates that health care is delivered in accordance with known best practice.

Health service research (HSR)

HSR is work that aims to generate new knowledge and understanding. The results must be generalisable and often play a key role in establishing evidence for best practice.

Clinical governance (CG)

CG is a framework through which NHS organisations are accountable for continuously improving the quality of their services and safeguarding high standards of care by creating an environment in which excellence in clinical care will flourish.

History

There have been many changes concerning health and social care provision over the last decade. In particular the political arena has seen rapid change since 1997, which culminated in the publication of *The NHS Plan – A Plan for Investment, A Plan for Reform* in July 2000 [2], the devolved versions being *Improving Health in Wales* in July 2001 [3] and *Pharmacy in Scotland – Creating an Integrated, Modern and Effective Health Service* in June 2001 [4]. Advancing technologies in surgical and medical care have provided choice for newer, questionably better and often more expensive answers to the population's ailments. A social evolution has also occurred where patients are encouraged to be participants and take more responsibility for their own health [5, 6]. These growing demands and expectations have led to a situation where the NHS must look for new ways of funding itself, of reducing costs and ultimately of making choices between health care projects and priorities. To make these difficult decisions, health care planners and policy-makers require information about the needs of their population, service provision and the extent to which the services meet the needs and the costs involved. With the advent of CG, practitioners are required to examine the systems which underpin the delivery of care in order to improve clinical care and the management of clinical risk is now high on all health care agendas [7, 8]. CG depends on the provision and understanding of evidence regarding the quality of clinical care being provided and must therefore be supported by robust, reliable research-based data. All these changes have intimately affected how health care professionals and their managers now view the NHS and research undertaken within it and has led to an expansion in HSR. Changing priorities in health care have not only encouraged refinements in established research methodologies such as randomised controlled trials (RCTs), case studies and surveys, but have also stimulated the development of new techniques, such as the use of quality indicators, meta-analysis and economic approaches to the evaluation of health care.

The Royal Pharmaceutical Society of Great Britain (RPSGB) recognised the need to develop strategic direction in PPR if pharmacy was to pursue a wider health care role. The momentum behind PPR was assisted by the Department of Health Enterprise Scheme in 1994 which provided funds for pharmacists to undertake projects in collaboration with other disciplines [9]. The RPSGB initiative Pharmacy In A New Age (PIANA) consolidated PPR as an independent discipline and identified five areas of research:

1. Managing minor ailments
2. Promoting and supporting healthy lifestyles
3. Managing prescribed medicines
4. Managing chronic conditions
5. Advising and supporting other health care professionals.

Three documents were produced from this scheme under the banners of *Pharmacy Practice: Setting the Research Agenda. Self-care and Pharmacy*; *Drug Therapy and Pharmacy*; *Pharmacist and the Profession* [10–12]. As part of the PIANA initiative, a pharmacy practice research and development task force was established to review the current status of PPR and to consider its future role. Four strategic goals were identified:

1. The research agenda in PPR should address the critical questions and health care priorities.
2. The research outputs in PPR should consistently meet generally accepted quality criteria.
3. An evaluative culture should be fostered within pharmacy practice.
4. PPR should be adequately and appropriately financed for the role required for it.

The task force also identified the need to address getting research into practice and set up a working party, which produced its report in February 1999 [13] and subsequently *Medicines, Pharmacy and the NHS: Getting it Right for Patients and Prescribers* in July 1999 [14]. Other documents that influenced the development of PPR included the Crown Review [15], initiated to determine in what circumstances health professionals could undertake new roles with regard to prescribing and supply of medicines in the course of their clinical practice [16], and *The Data Protection Act* of 1984 and 1998 [17, 18], regulating the processing of personal data and covering any storage system structure. In addition, the *Clinical Trials Directive* (draft) was introduced by the European Union to ensure good clinical and manufacturing practice in the preparation and manufacture of clinical trial materials.

Project design

Introduction

The design of a project can be described as a linear process. It starts with an initial research question, followed by a literature search and subsequently the choice of an appropriate research methodology which will allow the collection and presentation of data in the format required. However, what actually happens is a dynamic process (Figure 12.1). The original question will invariably be modified following literature searching, communication with experts in that field and methodological considerations such as 'is it feasible?' and 'does it produce the findings in the format I need?' Several cycles of this decision tree may be required before finalising the project design. Consideration should also be given to building a suitable team to facilitate and carry out the research. If statistical advice is required, this should also be sought at the design stage.

The research question

Questions generally arise if there is a discrepancy between what we know and what we would like to know and can come from any aspect of practice. However, research is more likely to be successful if the question is clear and precise. We may simply start with an interest in a particular area of research, which must be channelled into a general, and then more specific, research question. The question should be single and unambiguous, specific and appropriate and include the major elements of the investigation. The object of most HSR is to generate evidence about a particular practice or service. However, before proceeding any further, it is important to elucidate if this work has been done before. This involves carrying out a literature search and communicating with experts in the particular field to obtain current knowledge and trends of thought.

Literature search

Literature searching endeavours to access all relevant published literature on the chosen topic [19]. The worldwide web allows an individual to access an enormous amount of information. Although the internet has obvious advantages, it may still be necessary to develop the skills required to extract the appropriate information from the largest haystack imaginable! A practice researcher may look to employ the skills of a trained librarian to assist in this process.

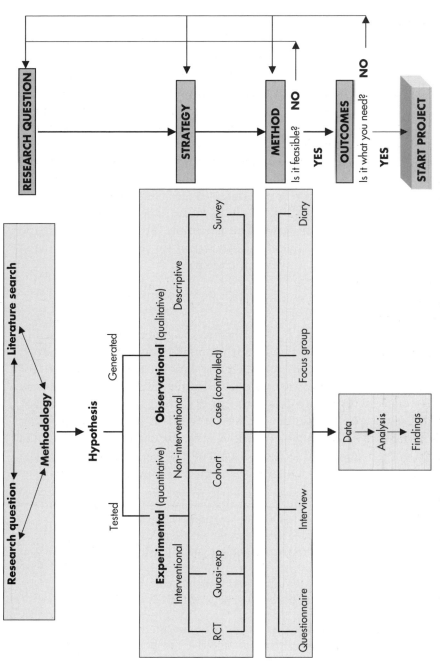

Figure 12.1 Project design decision tree. RCT, randomised controlled trial.

Search engines (e.g. www.google.com) are specific sites to help you browse or search for information on a particular subject. Gateways (e.g. www.biome.ac.uk – health and biomedical sciences) are central websites through which access to selected and evaluated sites may be gained, where Resource Discovery Network (www.rdn.ac.uk) will help you find the appropriate gateway. The literature search may provide evidence to answer the originally posed question or it may allow a hypothesis to be proposed. However, simply because an article is in print does not mean it contains accurate information. It is important to acknowledge the level of peer review assigned to an article and to be aware that anyone can publish on the internet. A process of critically appraising the article must therefore be carried out. This involves assessing results and interpreted conclusions in the light of the research design described and the appropriateness of that methodology to answer the question posed. Systematic reviews are a reliable source of information that use explicit and rigorous methods systematically to locate, appraise and synthesise evidence on a particular topic. The Cochrane database of systematic reviews and DARE (Database of Abstracts of Reviews of Effectiveness) are useful sites for finding systematic reviews.

Methodology

The research strategy can be described as the general approach used to address the research question, for example, an RCT or a survey, whereas the technique used to collect the data is called the method, for example, a questionnaire or interview (Figure 12.1). The method may be associated with certain design strategies such as surveys being carried out by structured questionnaires; however this is not a necessary link and any research strategy can be used with any method. Choosing the appropriate strategy and method is a balance between selecting the ideal design (highest validity) with the most practical (highest feasibility). Key points to decide are:

- Is there a hypothesis to test already (experimental/quantitative)?
- Is the aim to generate the hypothesis (observational/qualitative)?
- Is an experimental intervention going to be applied (interventional or non-interventional)?
- Are the data collected retrospectively from the past?
- Is the sample followed forward in time prospectively?

Methodologies can be described as either experimental or observational in nature (Figure 12.1).

Experimental studies usually involve measuring the effects that manipulating one variable has on another variable, for example in an RCT, and are considered a quantitative approach to research. Usually a hypothesis is tested using a random selection of samples from a known population. These samples are allocated to different experimental conditions where a small number of variables are measured and all other variables controlled. Statistics are usually applied to address internal validity (has the selected factor actually caused the effect seen?) and external validity (how generalisable are the data?). However, in practice research, random sampling of a known population is extremely difficult and the approach of quasi-experimentation has been developed. These experimental designs are more realistic for practice settings and consist of a wide range of methods, including, for example, comparisons of intact groups (such as patients attending a particular clinic) rather than random selection of samples.

Observational studies are usually more qualitative in approach where findings from an observation are described in words rather than numbers. This approach can be useful in areas where there is little pre-existing knowledge or when the issues are complex and require indepth exploration. Participatory observation is where the observer seeks to become a member of the group, and is largely qualitative, whereas structured observation can be more quantitative in style. These two approaches may be mixed to suit the required situation. Observational studies can be very time-consuming. They are also prone to confounding – this is where an apparent relationship is seen (or a real relationship is masked) but another factor has caused the effect, rather than the factor being tested.

Sometimes methodologies cannot be described in discrete entities and it may be more appropriate to use a hybrid approach (falling somewhere between the ideal methods) or a combination (linking two methods) to answer the posed question.

Case-control and cohort studies follow a quantitative, observational approach where intensive knowledge about a single case or small number of related cases is studied in their context. The data are collected using a range of techniques and provide evidence on patterns of disease occurrence in human populations and influential factors. A case-control study usually makes comparisons between a group of people who have the condition (the study group) and a group who do not (the control group). The control group is chosen to be as similar to the study group as possible but without the condition being investigated. Case-control studies can be relatively cheap and easy to run;

however they only test (rather than generate) a hypothesis and results can be difficult to interpret.

Cohort studies are concerned with following up a group of people over time and recording any changes that occur during this period. They can be expensive to run and are prone to bias and confounding factors. Case studies may involve both qualitative and quantitative tools where the dynamics of a single unit (person, organisation, etc.) are explored in depth over time.

Survey studies collect information in a standardised form from groups of people. They usually employ questionnaires or structured interviews to obtain a small amount of data from a large population. They tend to be well suited to descriptive studies, where there are no control groups; however they may be used to collect quantitative data. They can be cross-sectional (a snapshot of what is happening at one point in time) or longitudinal (looking at change or development over a period of time). Self-completed questionnaires are very efficient in terms of researchers' time and effort; however there is little check on the honesty of a response. Closed questions will provide more concise replies, but it is important to use careful wording. Open questions will need to be analysed, often by coding. This is a skilled and time-consuming process. Unstructured interviews are key tools for qualitative researchers where rich and indepth information is required from one person or a group of people (focus groups). Diaries are a kind of self-administered questionnaire where the process can range from being totally unstructured to a set of responses to specific questions. Scales and tests can be used to quantify an individual's performance or attitude to a particular situation. Attitude measurement is best achieved using a triangulation method of asking more than one question to gain an overall impression. A summated rating, or a Likert scale, is commonly used and is relatively easy to develop.

Ethics

Investigators must consider the ethical implications and psychological consequences for participants in their research and decide whether ethics approval is required. Early submission to the local research and ethics committee (LREC) is advisable to prevent the project experiencing a delayed start. All participants should have clear information on confidentiality, consent agreements and their right to withdraw from the research at any time. If a multicentred research project is to be undertaken approval must be sought from one of the regionally organised multicentre research ethics committees (MREC).

Funding

Funding is available from many sources (www.rdinfo.org.uk) [20, 21]. However, if a bid is to be successful, it must be appropriately targeted to the relevant body. There are four main categories of funding bodies: public sector; non-profit; private sector; and international. Examples of the public sector would include research councils such as the Medical Research Council, higher education authorities such as Scottish Higher Education funding council, government departments such as Welsh Office of Research and Development for Health and Social Care and a non-departmental public body such as the NHS Centre for Reviews and Dissemination. Non-profit sources of funding include charities such as the Wellcome Trust, Leverhulme Trust and King's Fund, professional bodies such as the Royal Pharmaceutical Society of Great Britain and schemes administered by universities and research institutes. The private sector consists of companies, e.g. pharmaceutical, that will fund research. European and international sources of funding include the European Commission, public bodies and foreign government and non-government bodies such as the World Health Organization. The Royal Pharmaceutical Society makes available a variety of grants and awards (www.rpsgb.org.uk). Annually the Practice Research Awards for practitioners in both hospital and community consist of the Galen Award (£10 000) and the Sir Hugh Linstead Community Research Fellowship (£12 000). Annual PhD studentships and intermittent awards relating to policy change are also available, e.g. professional development awards. The Guild of Healthcare Pharmacists is another body supportive of hospital pharmacy research. The majority of its awards tend to provide funding for presentation of completed work at conferences (www.ghp.org.uk). The UK Clinical Pharmacy Association also provides a variety of travel, training and conference attendance awards (www.ukcpa.org.uk). At individual trust level there are often in-house initiatives to support research which will be managed by the local research and development support unit. Government sources of funding will support policy developments and submissions should be aligned with local issues.

Dissemination

Dissemination of results is an essential part of the research process. The information must be publicly available and open to peer review so that assessment by professionals can create a consensus on acceptance into general practice.

Research can be disseminated in many ways, including full original peer-reviewed journal publications, oral and poster conference presentations, newsletters, reports or entry on to research databases. Publications are rewarding for researchers and not only raise their individual profile but also the profile of the profession in a multidisciplinary environment.

The future

The culture of evidence-based medicine has been established within the NHS; however the future now seems to be concerned with the delivery and the quality of that evidence. A *Research Governance Framework for Health and Social Care* was recently published by the Department of Health [22]. At the time of writing, this document only relates to England, although it will undoubtedly become a UK-wide programme and will ask researchers and colleagues to take responsibility for their activities in a similar way to the shift in clinical responsibility that has occurred through CG. The main aim of research governance is to encourage all NHS researchers to comply with a framework of activities and minimum standards and to be able to demonstrate their research quality through defined audit trails. However, there appears to be a rapidly changing agenda driven not only by the government and professional bodies, but also now by the patient. In the past, pharmacy research was primarily driven by professional and ethical requirements and in hospital was predominantly oriented towards pure science. With changing political agendas and increasing weight given to public opinion, pharmacy research has moved towards the social sciences and is more akin to general HSR. Here, I believe, a balance must be struck so as not to lose our professional skills to an ever-shifting government agenda. Amidst all the exciting changes within the NHS there has been difficulty in recruiting sufficient professionals to satisfy demand. This has challenged managers to find new ways of working. We must investigate and provide evidence to rectify these management issues so that our workforce for the future can meet the expectations of those from both within and outside the profession. Finally, the Medicines Management (MM) Collaborative has now gained momentum across England with several waves of community pilot sites working in multidisciplinary teams, showing how they can use their MM knowledge and skills to improve the care of patients [23]. Although this is a primary care venture, MM cuts across both the primary and secondary care structures and I believe the results from this venture will have broad implications for pharmacy service change.

References

1. RPSGB. *A New Age for Pharmacy Practice Research. Promoting Evidence-based Practice in Pharmacy*. London: RPSGB, 1997.
2. Department of Health. *The NHS Plan*. London: Department of Health, 2000.
3. National Assembly for Wales. *A Plan for the NHS with its Partners. Improving Health in Wales*. Cardiff: National Assembly for Wales, 2001.
4. RPSGB. *Creating an Integrated, Modern and Effective Health Service*. Edinburgh: Royal Pharmaceutical Society in Scotland, 2001.
5. RPSGB. *From Compliance to Concordance, Achieving Shared Goals in Medicine Taking*. London: RPSGB, 1997.
6. Department of Health. *Involving Patients and the Public in Healthcare. A Discussion Document*. London: Department of Health, 2001.
7. RPSGB. *Achieving Excellence in Pharmacy Through Clinical Governance*. London: RPSGB, 1999.
8. Department of Health. *A First Class Service: Quality in the New NHS*. London: Department of Health, 1999.
9. *The Pharmacy Practice Research Enterprise Scheme: A Resource Document*. Manchester: Pharmacy Practice Resource Centre, 1990.
10. RPSGB. *Pharmacy Practice: Setting the Research Agenda. Self-care and Pharmacy*. London: RPSGB, 1998.
11. RPSGB. *Pharmacy Practice: Setting the Research Agenda. Drug Therapy and Pharmacy*. London: RPSGB, 1998.
12. RPSGB. *Pharmacy Practice: Setting the Research Agenda. Pharmacy and the Profession*. London: RPSGB, 2001.
13. RPSGB. *Getting Research into Pharmacy Practice*. London: RPSGB, 1999.
14. RPSGB. *Medicines, Pharmacy and the NHS: Getting it Right for Patients and Prescribers. Setting the Clinical Effectiveness Agenda for Pharmacy*. London: RPSGB, 1999.
15. Department of Health. *Review of Prescribing, Supply and Administration of Medicines – A Report on the Supply and Administration of Medicines under Group Protocols*. London: Department of Health, 1998.
16. Department of Health. *Review of Prescribing, Supply and Administration of Medicines – Final Report*. London: Department of Health, 1999.
17. Department of Health. *The Data Protection Act*. London: Department of Health, 1998.
18. Wingfield J. The Data Protection Act 1998. *Pharm J* 2000; 265: 31.
19. Hart C. *Doing a Literature Review*. London: Sage, 1998.
20. Hawkes C, ed. *The Research Funding Guide*. London: Research Fortnight, 1998.
21. The Association of Medical Research Charities (UK). *The Association of Medical Research Charities Handbook*. Wigston: Chartwell Press, 2000.
22. Department of Health. *Research Governance Framework*. London: Department of Health, 2001.

23. Thompson M. Collaborative National Medicines Management Service seeks to spread good practice. *Pharm J* 2001; 266: 378.

Further reading

Greenhalgh T. *How to Read a Paper*. London: BMJ Publishing, 1997.

Hart C. *Doing a Literature Review*. London: Sage, 2000.

Oppenheim A N. *Questionnaire Design, Interviewing and Attitude Measurement*. London: Cassell, 1992.

Robson C. *Real World Research*, 2nd edn. Oxford: Blackwell, 2002.

Smith F. *Research Methods in Pharmacy Practice*. London: Pharmaceutical Press, 2001.

Wiffen P. *Evidence-based Pharmacy*. Oxford: Radcliffe Medical Press, 2001.

13

Education and training

Trevor Beswick and Lynne Bollington

Appropriate education and training is the key issue for any health care professional, in terms of providing a competent, effective, efficient and high-quality service to patients. Though moves towards multiprofessional education and training are being made, for most health care professionals, it is undertaken on a unidisciplinary and uniprofessional basis. In terms of postregistration training, it is often the service itself that provides the strategic direction for training and the degree to which it supports service development.

As a professional group, hospital pharmacists in the UK have made reasonable progress in the way that they have used training to underpin changing services and roles. One should not be complacent and there are always opportunities to improve, but many of the elements of hospital pharmacy service as currently practised would not be in place without appropriate training of pharmacists, pharmacy technicians and assistants.

History

One of the fundamental changes in roles took place in the 1960s and 1970s with the introduction of ward pharmacy services. These services were developed at a time when many traditional preparative roles in hospital were being absorbed by the pharmaceutical industry. Through the 1980s clinical pharmacy services became more widespread and more accomplished and started to reflect the aspirations of the concept of 'pharmaceutical care', as described by Hepler and Strand [1]. The fact that the hospital pharmacist has a key role in the individualisation of drug treatment in patients as well as a strategic role in managing medicines at an organisational level was formally recognised by the Department of Health in England in 1988 (HC(88)54) [2]. These changes were covered in more depth in chapter 7.

During this time, a number of postregistration courses were developed; these ranged from short courses through to fully taught MSc degrees. They had the common aim of improving hospital pharmacists' effectiveness in contributing to the care of patients, through applying their knowledge of pharmacology and pharmaceutics to the care of patients. A key skill that needed development was that of being able to work with the rest of the health care team and, in particular, good communication skills.

Alongside the development of the pharmacists' roles came the need to make better use of pharmacy technicians. With increasing use of computers in dispensaries, decentralisation of supply functions (ward top-up) and more aseptic preparative work of intravenous products there were great opportunities for pharmacy technicians and assistants. These developments were also driven by chief pharmacists needing to maximise their productivity during times of increasing workloads and constrained funding by using the most appropriate skill-mix within their departments. Again, bringing staff into new roles could not be accomplished without training. In the 1990s, the increasing importance of the whole issue of risk management gave another focus for the need for training. Service providers needed to demonstrate that staff were trained, and trained properly (accredited), to undertake the roles that they undertook. This became particularly important in the context of aseptic preparative services in the mid-1990s.

The 1990s saw the introduction of competency-based training schemes for pharmacy technicians and for preregistration pharmacists. In the case of pharmacy technicians, this move was driven by the educational sector and was part of a general move to develop vocational training schemes that were more focused on occupational competencies rather than knowledge per se.

In the late 1990s, the new Labour government brought a heightened focus on service quality to the National Health Service (NHS). Its paper *A First Class Service* brought forward the concepts of clinical governance and lifelong learning [3]. These identified that appropriate training of staff should be provided, as well as promoting systems to ensure that their continued professional development needs are met. Further emphasis on skill-mix, multiprofessional working, better use of information technology and automation as well as a wish to disregard many old interprofessional boundaries once again brought opportunities for the development of new roles. As a consequence we see pharmacists becoming more clinically specialised (likely to take on prescribing roles), pharmacy technicians (with greater responsibility for dispensing) taking on more responsibilities and pharmacy assistants moving more and more into mainstream hospital pharmacy work. The Audit Commission as well as the Controls Assurance Standards emphasise the need for appropriate training for those dealing with medicines [4, 5].

The present day

Undergraduate and preregistration

Currently, 16 universities in the UK offer pharmacy degree courses. Since 1997, pharmacy has been a 4-year course, leading to the MPharm degree. Two universities offer sandwich courses delivered over 5 years, incorporating the preregistration year. The first graduates from the MPharm degree left university in summer 2001 to take up preregistration training positions. In recognition of the need for greater numbers of pharmacists to undertake new roles and provide a greater range of pharmacy services, most universities have increased their intake of students, and in addition two new sites have recently become accredited.

To become a pharmacist, all graduates must complete a 1-year period of preregistration training under the supervision of a registered pharmacist. In addition, all trainees must pass a registration examination. The Royal Pharmaceutical Society of Great Britain (RPSGB) sets the standards for the training, and monitors the quality to ensure that it is acceptably high across all sites.

A full revision of the preregistration training programme was undertaken by the RPSGB in preparation for the intake of the first graduates from the new 4-year degree in August 2001. The aim of the new training programme was to develop pharmacists who had patients as their primary focus and who were fit for practice in any sector of the profession. Putting patients at the centre of care was a clear theme within *Pharmacy in the Future*, the document dealing with pharmacy's part in the NHS Plan, so the change in focus was timely [6]. One of the major changes that was implemented to achieve fitness for practice in all sectors was the requirement for all graduates to undertake some period of their training in both hospital and community pharmacy.

The new training programme comprises performance standards which state what a newly qualified pharmacist is expected to be able to do. These were devised in consultation with members of all sectors of the profession and describe generic skills required of all pharmacists. The examination syllabus was revised and updated, and now has a stronger emphasis on the ability of pharmacists to perform calculations.

The shift to a more outcome-focused programme enables preregistration trainees to assess themselves against the performance standards and so identify what their learning needs are, hence reinforcing the culture of continuing professional development (CPD) that is being developed throughout the profession. In tandem with the trainee, preregistration tutors also have to demonstrate a commitment to CPD and maintain a portfolio in which they document how they have identified and met their learning needs. Table 13.1 gives some definitions that should help to clarify terms used in this chapter.

The vast majority of hospital trainees undergo an in-house training programme that typically consists of a planned rotation through the main sections within the pharmacy department. This will often include periods in the dispensary, wards and clinical services, medicines information, technical services and quality assurance. Depending on the size of the hospital and the scope of services offered, there might well be a period of training at a neighbouring hospital for specialist experience. Most in-house training programmes are supplemented by a programme of regionally taught courses, which may be delivered either as 1-day courses or as residential blocks.

Students undergo formal assessments with their tutor during the year, and the results of these are sent to the RPSGB. In addition, the RPSGB requests copies of the in-house and taught course programmes, and may sample the tutor portfolios to enable closer monitoring of the quality of training.

Table 13.1 Definitions in education and training

Term	Definition
Continuing education	Taking opportunities to learn that are relevant to current or future roles. Usually a formal course or educational package
Continuing professional development (CPD)	The broader aspects of learning and developing, including training, learning lessons in a working environment and gaining insights into professional practice
Reflective practice	The approach to development whereby an individual thinks through events and experiences (what went well, what went badly) to improve practice
Lifelong learning	CPD plus all other aspects of personal learning, including those outside the work context

Pharmacists

Hospital pharmacist training continues after qualification. Currently there is a structured grading system in place (see chapter 1); A-, B- and many C-grade pharmacist posts are designated as training grades. Typically, trainees will move through a programme of in-house rotational experience, reinforcing the experience gained as a preregistration trainee. In addition, formalised training opportunities are available for all grades of staff to suit their level of experience or their specialisation.

The majority of newly qualified hospital pharmacists undertake postgraduate diplomas or masters degrees in topics such as clinical pharmacy or technical services, although a wide range of postgraduate courses exist and can be undertaken at any stage in a pharmacist's career [7]. The qualifications tend to be offered either as a taught course or as a distance-learning package, usually linked to work-based practice experience, such as contributions made to patient interventions or attending clinical rounds.

Some pharmacists choose to undertake a course specifically related to their area of pharmacy practice (e.g. medicines information, clinical pharmacy teaching or radiopharmacy) or to their clinical speciality (for example, psychiatric pharmacy). Others choose to undertake a multidisciplinary programme, such as a management course.

Many universities have encouraged people to undertake more postgraduate education by enabling flexible progression though modularised courses. Often the modules can be accrued over a number of years, and the student can gain credits towards a qualification at certificate, diploma, masters or DPharm level.

As well as the opportunities for gaining formalised qualifications, opportunities for accessing general continuing education are well supported for hospital pharmacy staff.

Most regional education providers run programmes of taught courses on current topics and therapeutic updates. These are often supplemented locally by in-house educational meetings and evening events run by organisations such as the Guild of Healthcare Pharmacists, the RPSGB local branches and the Centres for Pharmacy Postgraduate Education (see chapter 15 for information on support organisations).

More recently there have been moves to develop competency-based schemes for clinical pharmacists [8, 9]. Rather than just ensuring the pharmacists have a good knowledge base, these schemes begin to identify the skills needed to provide pharmaceutical care and attempt to demonstrate that the skills and knowledge are applied in practice, not just for a course or in an examination setting.

There has always been strong support for continuing education within the hospital service, and more recently as the culture shifts towards CPD, efforts are being made to facilitate CPD within the workplace.

Technician training

Student technician training has evolved dramatically over recent years, since the introduction of the National Vocational Qualification (NVQ) Level 3 in Pharmacy Services in 1997. This is a competency-based training programme, consisting of a total of nine (seven core and two optional) units that the student undertakes in the workplace. The student must demonstrate consistent competence in a range of activities, and undergoes assessment by local work-based tutors. The tutors must gain D32/33 qualifications that help to ensure that they are able to judge evidence fairly and consistently [10].

In addition to the work-based units, students must also gain evidence of their underpinning knowledge. This may be achieved in several ways – some hospitals use distance-learning packages, such as those provided by the National Pharmaceutical Association (NPA) or the Buttercups scheme. Others attend local BTEC colleges for the underpinning knowledge teaching. Revised standards for NVQ level 3 were introduced in September 2002.

Until recently the opportunities for structured postqualification training for technicians were very limited. However, over the last 2–3 years, as technicians have begun to move into new roles within the pharmacy department and take on additional responsibilities, the need for formal training and accreditation to perform these new roles has been increasingly recognised.

The first major development for technician training was the introduction of technician checking schemes, which have allowed technicians to perform the final accuracy check of dispensed items. Most NHS regions have now developed accredited schemes that specify the training that an individual must undergo, and the mechanisms for assessment [11]. Upon completion of all stages they gain formal accreditation, which can be recognised by other NHS employers.

Pharmacy technicians are now developing into other roles, particularly working more closely with patients and performing medicines management roles. New schemes that will enable accreditation of technicians in medicines management and medicines information are currently being developed. The South East South Coast education team's Medication Management course, aimed at supporting technicians who work with a patient's own drugs scheme, is an example of this (Goodson *et al.*, personal communication).

Support staff

In tandem with the developing roles of pharmacists and pharmacy technicians, efforts are being made to ensure that pharmacy assistants are given appropriate support to underpin the roles that they are now performing within the pharmacy. In recognition of this, training programmes to support and accredit these roles are being developed at a local and regional level. At the time of writing, a national qualification, in the form of an NVQ level 2, is anticipated for pharmacy assistants.

Management and leadership

The Audit Commission makes it clear that excellent pharmacy services require good leadership [4]. Development of management and leadership skills in pharmacy is therefore an important aspect of CPD. Chapter 14 deals with the key aspects of management; this chapter will briefly mention some important training initiatives. Often the first aspects of management training will be taught in the local hospital on a multiprofessional basis – personnel management, understanding the organisation, budget control, for example. Access to external training may be provided, such as to the Open University health management courses or to Masters in Business Administration (MBA), for those taking on full-time management roles. The national development scheme for senior pharmacists, and the more recently introduced national course for technicians, is an invaluable opportunity to gain insight and develop skills in a uniprofessional setting [12, 13]. Within the West Midlands a pharmacy management programme has been developed in conjunction with Aston University to ensure that future managers are equipped for their roles [14].

The future

The NHS will continue to modernise and change. This will bring new demands on the profession that will need to be underpinned with well-educated, trained and competent staff.

Pharmacists will need training and accreditation if prescribing roles are to be developed and will represent a quantum change in the training of pharmacists. In time we can expect that such training will form part of the undergraduate course that in itself may develop to include more practice-based experience and multiprofessional work.

The increasing importance of CPD and a link, through mandatory CPD, to registration will have a key impact on individual professionals. It will be their own responsibility, shared to a degree with their employer, to maintain appropriate competencies to practice by making use of a range of continuing education, reflective practice and experiential learning. There will be a need for more quality assurance of training, delivered through accreditation of courses and course providers. The quality of placements for preregistration training is already being assessed by commissioning groups (those funding placements – the Workforce Development Confederations) in addition to the RPSGB.

It is likely that, as their roles carry increasing responsibilities, pharmacy technicians will become a registered profession. This in itself will bring both challenges and opportunities to pharmacists. As pharmacists continue to develop specialised clinical roles there will need to be appropriate training and mechanisms for accreditation of individuals to perform those roles.

References

1. Hepler C D, Strand L M. Opportunities and responsibilities in pharmaceutical care. *Am J Hosp Pharm* 1990; 47: 533–543.
2. Department of Health. *The Way Forward for Hospital Pharmaceutical Services*. HC(88)54. London: Department of Health, 1988.
3. Department of Health. *A First Class Service: Quality in the New NHS*. London: The Stationery Office, 1998.
4. Audit Commission. *A Spoonful of Sugar – Managing Medicines in NHS Hospitals*. London: Audit Commission, 2001.
5. NHS Executive Controls Assurance Standard on Medicines Management, Revision 02 (October 2001) www.open.gov.uk/doh/riskman.htm (accessed 12 May 2002).
6. Department of Health. *Pharmacy in the Future – Implementing the NHS Plan*. London: Department of Health, 2000.
7. Anonymous. Formal postgraduate courses for practising pharmacists. *Pharm J* 2002; 268: 729–736.
8. Goldsmith G. *An Investigation of the Effect a Competency Based Training Programme has on Junior Pharmacists' Satisfaction and Fitness for Purpose*. MSc thesis. Brighton: University of Brighton, 2001.

9. McRobbie D, Webb D G, Bates I *et al.* Assessment of clinical competence: designing a competence grid for junior pharmacists. *Pharm Ed* 2001; 1: 67–76.
10. Culshaw M, Hemingway L. Assessing the assessors for NVQ awards – the D32/D33 experience. *Pharm Manage* 1996; 12: 2–3.
11. Evans D, O'Loan L. The North Thames pharmacy accredited checking technician (ACT) scheme. *CPD Pharm* 2000; 1: 7–11.
12. www.gouldwa.freeserve.co.uk/Ndssp/course.html National development scheme for senior pharmacists (accessed 18 May 2002).
13. www.gouldwa.freeserve.co.uk/Ndsspt/course.html National development scheme for senior pharmacy technicians (accessed 18 May 2002).
14. Bassan S S, Marriot J. Hospital Pharmacy Management Diploma – the first year. *Hosp Pharm* 1999; 6: 173–175.

Further reading

Brackley K, Evans D, Haria M *et al.* Developing CPD in the workplace: the implementation of a regional support strategy. *Pharm J* 2002; 268: 726–728.
Formal postgraduate courses for practising pharmacists. *Pharm J* 2002; 268: 729–736.
Purkiss R. Reflective practice. *Pharm Manage* 2002; 18: 8–10.

14

Managing services

Pippa Roberts and Peter Sharott

Preregistration trainees and newly registered pharmacists entering hospital pharmacy may have given little consideration to their potential future roles as managers. At these early stages in their career, attention will be focused on gaining experience in the broad range of pharmacy services and having the opportunity to apply their knowledge to practical situations. Most pharmacists will have aspirations to work in a clinical setting where they are able to operate as part of a clinical team, directly contributing to the management and care of patients.

At this stage pharmacists are dependent on their managers to provide them with training opportunities, guidance and support. There will be a reasonable expectation that their managers will be experienced, knowledgeable and accessible, and able to provide a continuous and dependable source of ready-made solutions to problems they encounter. They will probably have little appreciation of the wide range of skills that their managers have acquired and are using for their benefit.

Progression up the career ladder, beyond the training grades, will lead to posts, particularly at grade C and D level, with an increasing management component, involving staff management and responsibility for a section of the service. This is the stage when pharmacists acquire the ability to balance managerial responsibility with the stimulation of working in a clinical setting, whilst maintaining high professional standards and judgement.

This chapter is intended to provide an insight into and appreciation of the roles pharmacy managers undertake within the pharmacy department and how they interact with other managers in the wider hospital environment.

Pharmacy management

The National Health Service (NHS) is sometimes criticised for employing excessive numbers of managers whose existence diverts resources away from front-line clinical services. In reality, hospitals are extremely complex organisations that depend on experienced, well-trained managers for the development and delivery of high-quality, efficient, patient-centred services. Hospital pharmacy departments, albeit on a much smaller scale, can also be very complex organisations, offering a wide selection of services provided by a professional, technical and support staff comprising as many as 150–200 people. Pharmacy managers, working at different levels in the department, make a critical contribution to patient care by applying a wide variety of skills, expertise and experience in the delivery and development of clinical and support services that are compatible with the overall aims of the hospital.

Ultimate managerial responsibility for the pharmacy service will rest with the NHS trust's chief pharmacist who will be accountable to a senior manager, often one of the executive directors. The chief pharmacist will also be accountable to the trust's board for all aspects of the safe storage, handling, distribution and use of all medicines throughout the hospital. This responsibility encompasses the need to ensure that all practice involving medicines complies with current legislation, NHS rules and regulations, such as the recently introduced Controls Assurance Standards and corporate governance, which incorporates a requirement for probity and financial control into all aspects of the organisation's day-to-day business. The chief pharmacist will also be responsible for pharmacy's contribution to the clinical governance agenda. This demands that all patients receive the highest possible standard of care, that practice is evidence-based and is delivered by appropriately trained and qualified staff, and that risks to patients during their treatment are minimised.

Effective management of pharmacy services demands high levels of leadership and teamwork. The chief pharmacist is not only required to lead the pharmacy service but also to act as an advocate for and representative of the service within the organisation as a whole. Responsibility for the pharmacy budget requires the ability to obtain sufficient resources to maintain and develop services; it is equally important that the service is able to function as part of the larger organisation and to respond to the introduction of new services arising from changing priorities.

The two broad types of management are generally referred to as operational and strategic management. Operational management focuses on the wide range of functions which underpin the day-to-day smooth running of the pharmacy department. Problems tend to be addressed as they occur through a pragmatic approach to decision-making. Strategic management, on the other hand, is associated with the need to identify future service developments and draw up plans which can deliver them. As staff progress up the management ladder there should be an increasing shift away from substantially operational management to a significant element of strategic management. Hence, the strategic management role performed by the chief pharmacist should receive far more emphasis and time, while operational matters are delegated to more junior staff. Such delegation is not only important to the chief pharmacist, but also ensures that subordinates can take a large measure of responsibility for their services and are fully tested in their management role. It is critical that the chief pharmacist has a vision about the future direction of the pharmacy service and can draw up plans for changing the delivery of services, making better use of staff and obtaining resources to upgrade or replace equipment and facilities. However, this strategic role will not be the exclusive province of the chief pharmacist as the entire management team should be able to contribute to the generation of new ideas and the production of specific plans for their own areas of responsibility.

This chief pharmacist's leadership role will be supported by a team of senior pharmacists and technicians who take responsibility for major sections of the department, such as patient services, clinical pharmacy services, medicines information, aseptic dispensing, non-sterile and sterile production, quality assurance, procurement and stores. Such managers need to acquire a wide range of skills and expertise. Staff will have the opportunity to attend a wide range of training courses in order to develop their management skills, but there is no substitute for gaining experience and developing expertise through performing the job.

A particularly positive development has been the increasing number of pharmacy technicians who now hold senior management positions. This recognises the significant contribution that technicians can make to managing key sections of the department, such as the dispensary, procurement, stores and distribution, and is an important means of providing technicians with improved prospects for career progression. There is also the added significant benefit of allowing pharmacists to concentrate on the management and development of clinical and patient-centred pharmacy services.

In summary, chief pharmacists and their senior management team hold considerable power insomuch that they have the ability to determine, negotiate and implement the future direction of the pharmacy service. Not only will a strong management team be able to make the best use of staff and resources, it will also be able to exert a strong influence beyond the confines of the pharmacy department in achieving a high profile for the service.

Business planning

An NHS trust is essentially a non-profit-making business whose chief executive and board are accountable for delivering high, safe standards of care for its patients through the effective and efficient use of resources within an agreed annual budget. Each year all NHS organisations are required to undertake an extensive and detailed business planning exercise. Within each NHS trust the business planning process is intended to identify anticipated changes in the provision of services and to define its ability to respond to changing priorities determined by local and national policies. For example, implementation of key government policies affecting the care of older patients and patients with cancer and coronary heart disease may require the introduction of new, extended or redesigned services in order to meet agreed performance targets.

For an NHS trust the primary objective of the business planning process is to ensure that sufficient income is gained from local commissioning bodies – the primary care trusts – to cover the full cost of providing services. This requires the construction of budgets that take account of planned changes in clinical activity and case mix. Funding must cover staff salaries and overheads, non-staff expenditure, such as estate and utility costs, and the revenue consequences of capital developments. Capital funding itself, required for the purchase of new equipment and the construction of new or refurbished facilities, will be obtained either from a block allocation or by specific business cases.

Within the organisation, an NHS trust will normally devolve the budget to the individual clinical and non-clinical directorates. The directorate managers will have responsibility for managing their budgets and for developing their own business plans and constructing budgets to cover their services.

In business planning terms, the pharmacy department is a cog in the trust's big wheel. The chief pharmacist will be required to produce an annual business plan which meets the changing requirements and service objectives of the clinical directorates as well as the organisation as a whole. The crucial role of the chief pharmacist, supported by the rest of the pharmacy management team, is to act as an advocate for the pharmacy service and ensure that sufficient resources are available to maintain and develop services in line with the overall direction and objectives of the directorates and the trust. This will invariably require the application of considerable negotiating skills to secure an appropriate share of limited resources. The main objective will be to ensure that the pharmacy department is able to secure sufficient resources to maintain safe and effective services and to minimise risk to patients through the provision of appropriate clinical services. As new hospital services are identified and developed, the chief pharmacist will need to ensure that their impact on the pharmacy service has been properly assessed and, where appropriate, additional resources allocated. Although a proactive approach to service development may sometimes lead to failure and disappointment, success is more likely to be achieved when pharmacy managers recognise that strategic planning is a vital support mechanism for maintaining a dynamic and forward-moving service.

Preparing a business case

The business planning process is often underpinned by a requirement to prepare a detailed business case which provides a thorough analysis of the implications for changing or developing services. Not only will a business case be used to judge the merits of the specific proposal, it may also be compared with business cases from other departments or directorates as part of a prioritisation exercise. Pharmacy managers need, therefore, to muster all their skills, knowledge and expertise to produce a well-reasoned, robust case which can withstand detailed scrutiny.

In most business cases it is expected that a range of options will be described. These may range from the 'do nothing' approach to an option that requires the highest level of funding in terms of capital investment and revenue consequences. High-cost capital projects may require a bid for funding from an external source, such as one of the commissioning authorities or the Department of Health. The business case will need to be extremely well-argued, show a detailed financial analysis and, perhaps most importantly, educate and inform non-pharmacy managers and clinicians about the issues affecting the delivery of a modernised pharmacy service.

Budget management

The total annual budget for a hospital trust will be in the order of £100 million, though for large teaching trusts and merged organisations the figure may be several times larger. About 70% of the expenditure will be taken up in the costs of employing and paying staff. Drug expenditure will account for about 15–20% of the remaining non-staff expenditure. This represents about £4.5–5m a year for a local district general hospital but will be nearer £20m a year for a large specialised teaching hospital. Not surprisingly, managing and controlling drug expenditure is often given high priority by hospital managers because of the potential to make significant cost savings and the risk from failure to stay within predetermined budgets.

A key responsibility for the chief pharmacist is management of the pharmacy budget. The vast majority of the budget will be the recurring revenue cost of employing staff. The remainder of the pharmacy budget will cover non-staff expenditure, such as containers and other disposables, labels and the maintenance of equipment. There may also be a capital budget for the purchase of new equipment. Although most pharmacy budgets no longer include the main drug budgets for the hospital, they may cover the purchase of medical gases and products used in clinical support departments.

All budgets will be set on an annual basis, although some changes may be incorporated during the financial year, particularly where changes to staffing levels have been agreed. The chief pharmacist, as the budget holder, will be expected to ensure that expenditure does not exceed the agreed budget.

Staffing budget

A typical NHS trust, managing a small district general hospital (DGH), will employ about 40 pharmacy staff covering a range of staff groups. Larger trusts, with a large DGH or two or more smaller DGHs, will have up to 80 pharmacy staff, while teaching hospitals may have over 150 staff. The staffing establishment will comprise professional, technical, ancillary and administrative and clerical staff, as well as pharmacist and technician trainees. As often staff work on a part-time basis, the number of people employed, known as the headcount, will generally exceed the number of established whole-time-equivalent posts (WTEs).

Typically, about 40% of the pharmacy staff will be pharmacists, 30% will be technicians, 15% will be ancillary and 8% administrative and clerical staff. A further 8% of the staff will be either preregistration trainees or technician trainees. A ratio of $1:1:1$ (pharmacist : technicians : others) has been suggested as an appropriate balance [1].

The final staffing budget will be calculated on the agreed staffing establishment for the department measured as WTEs. The budget will reflect the grades, salaries and allowances, such as London weighting and emergency duty commitments, for each staff member, and will also include the employer's overhead costs, such as national insurance and superannuation (pension) payments.

In a typical pharmacy with a staff of 40 WTEs, the annual staffing budget will be in the order of £800 000. Departments with 150 WTEs will have an annual budget of about £3.5m.

When managers experience difficulty in filling vacant posts on a long-term, permanent basis they are often obliged to rely on the availability of temporary staff supplied by locum agencies. Such staff are more expensive than permanent staff and present a particular challenge for budget management. In practice, this means that it is not always possible to employ sufficient locum staff to cover all vacant posts, thus placing an additional strain on the department's ability to maintain a full range of services.

Drug budgets

In the past, drug budgets formed the majority of the pharmacy budget and were the responsibility of the chief pharmacist. Today, in most trusts each clinical directorate is accountable for managing its own drug budget. The directorate drug budgets will probably be further subdivided to each of their clinical subspecialities. For example, in a medicine directorate there may be subspecialities for cardiology, dermatology, gastroenterology and elderly services.

Despite devolvement of the drug budgets, pharmacists continue to play a pivotal role in setting and monitoring the budgets and producing regular reports on expenditure.

The directorate pharmacists will be in the best position to provide ongoing advice to directorate managers and clinicians on achieving effective management of drug budgets without compromising patient care. Using data from the pharmacy's computer system they can produce regular reports to monitor drug expenditure against the agreed budget. If expenditure begins to exceed the budget they can identify the drugs that are having the greatest impact and propose possible remedial action. In practice, it is not always easy to maintain effective budget control as factors such as changing clinical case mix, increased through-put of patients and isolated use of expensive treatments on a small number of patients may have a disproportionate but significant impact on overall expenditure trends. Successful management of drug expenditure should also be seen in the context of the trust's medicines management system, including control of available drugs through the formulary and the process for managing the introduction of new drugs (see chapter 8). A particularly relevant management role is the use of efficient and effective medicines procurement and stock control systems that minimise acquisition costs and wastage (see chapter 1).

As part of a trust's annual business planning process, pharmacy managers, in collaboration with their directorate pharmacists, should be involved in the estimation of drug budgets for the forthcoming year. The primary purpose of this exercise will be to set budgets that have been adjusted for the impact of a variety of critical factors and influences. These may include anticipated changes in clinical activity and case mix, the potential impact of new – invariably more expensive – recently licensed drugs, changes in drug treatment preferences, savings from negotiated purchasing contracts and, conversely, increases in the acquisition costs of medicines. Although it would be extremely difficult to achieve total accuracy in the budget-setting process, it is important to achieve a level of confidence in the budgets, particularly from the consultants, so that a greater commitment to effective expenditure control can be maintained during the financial year. This level of control is seen as a performance target for trusts [2].

Benchmarking

Managers working at all levels of the organisation have an obligation to ensure that their services are constantly reviewed and are adapted to meet the changing needs of patients and staff. In the NHS, benchmarking has become increasingly recognised as a valuable management tool for assessing the performance of a service and identifying opportunities for developing better services and using staff more effectively and efficiently [3, 4]. An important feature of benchmarking is comparison with other similar-sized hospitals or services, as this allows managers to consider alternative ways of planning and delivering their services based on the wider experience of others.

The primary aim of a benchmarking exercise is to use and collect data to provide quantitative and, preferably, qualitative means of measuring performance through the production of a range of indicators, which can be compared with other similar organisations. Ideally, benchmarks should be sufficiently sensitive to demonstrate whether gaps in service provision may lead to less effective medicines management and increased risk for patients. For example, the lack of enough trained, experienced clinical pharmacists may reduce the quality of prescription intervention monitoring, as well as providing insufficient prescribing support for the junior doctors. Within the pharmacy department, an inadequate staffing establishment required to manage the dispensing workloads may cause increased error rates.

As previously discussed, the hospital pharmacy service is characterised by the number of posts in the staffing establishment, measured as WTEs. The establishment will comprise professional, technical, ancillary and administrative and clerical staff, as well as pharmacist and technician trainees. The numbers, grades and types of staff employed are commonly referred to as the skill-mix. The process of reviewing the composition and size of the staffing establishment is known as manpower planning. The other way of characterising the pharmacy service is in terms of the range of services provided and the numbers, grades and types of staff employed in each section. The ultimate aim should be to achieve a staffing establishment and skill-mix in the department that correlate with the size, complexity and clinical activity of the hospital and the demands and workloads placed on the pharmacy service.

Benchmarks for pharmacy are produced by combining the clinical activity, workload data and staffing information to produce indicators such as the number of staff per 1000 inpatient bed days or 1000 outpatient attendances. These indicators can then be used both to compare different hospitals and to produce annual trend data for an individual hospital.

In December 2001 the Audit Commission published its comprehensive report, entitled A *Spoonful of Sugar*, on medicines management in NHS hospitals [2]. The report provides an indepth review of over 200 acute NHS trusts in England and Wales and has 33 recommendations for improving the ways in which organisations manage medicines and deliver pharmacy services. In essence, this work has for the first time generated an extensive database and a range of indicators that can be used to compare the performance of NHS trusts.

From a manager's viewpoint the Audit Commission's report provides an opportunity to take pharmacy services benchmarking to a new level, in terms of an ability to calculate the numbers and types of staff required to deliver a modern, patient-centred service. This will provide an opportunity to develop a vision for a pharmacy service based on

Table 14.1 Benchmarking: examples of criteria used to build up performance indicators

Trust clinical activity data	Staff (WTEs) and grade by pharmacy function and expenditure	Pharmacy activity and workload data	Pharmacy activity functions
Inpatient days	Pharmacists	Dispensed medicines	Aseptic services
Occupied-bed days	Preregistration trainees	• Inpatients	Clinical pharmacy
Finished consultant episodes	Pharmacy technicians	• Discharge	• Ward pharmacy
Day cases	Pharmacy technician trainees	• Outpatients	• Clinical directorate support
Outpatient attendances	Assistant technical officers	• A&E	• Clinical training
A&E attendances	Administrative and clerical	• Aseptic products	• Therapeutic drug monitoring
	Other grades	Medication errors	• Audit
	Total WTEs	• Administration	Community care support
	Total staff expenditure	• Dispensing	Computer and IT support
		• Prescribing	Dispensing
		Medicines information enquiries	• Inpatient and discharge
		Prescription interventions	• Outpatients
		Procurement order numbers	Drug distribution
		Ward pharmacy visits	Education and training provision
		Stockholdings	Formulary management
		Stock items issued	Management and administration
		Drug expenditure	Medicines information
		• Total expenditure	Procurement and stores
		• Inpatient expenditure	Production and repacking
		• Outpatient expenditure	

A&E, Accident and Emergency; WTEs, whole-time-equivalent posts; IT, information technology.

effective manpower planning and the extensive use of modern technology, such as electronic prescribing and automated dispensaries. Table 14.1 identifies a range of factors that can be used to build up benchmarking data.

Staff management

The management of people is probably the single most difficult aspect of management, at once being the most challenging, the most frustrating and the most exciting. It is the aspect of management that often receives the least attention, often regarded as common sense so not requiring special training or analysis. Whereas other aspects of managers' jobs are thought to require qualifications and training, the human aspect, competence in managing people, is all too frequently regarded as something that develops automatically without help; this could be a serious and potentially costly error. The starting point for staff management is selection.

Selection strategy

Every pharmacist with responsibility for recruitment from preregistration onwards needs to be skilled in staff selection. Pharmacists will have access to expert advice and assistance on policies and procedures from personnel departments, but they will not to take over the responsibilities of the employing manager. The pharmacy team's performance remains the responsibility of the chief pharmacist – getting the right people in the team is crucial to success.

Generally, when a managerial appointment is taken a team is inherited, so selection skills are only required when vacancies occur. Even so, the ability to choose the right person for the right job is essential. The following questions should be considered before the recruitment process begins, so that the manager has an idea of the general requirements of the team and then particular needs can be identified when advertising specific posts:

- What kind of team does the pharmacy department currently have?
- What kind of people does the pharmacy need to meet the departmental objectives?
- How many people does the pharmacy department need?
- What roles does the department need the individuals within the team to fulfil?
- What changes in team composition are required?
- What personal dynamics does the group entail?

Often an important source of information about the purpose and function of the pharmacy team comes from the job description and objectives of the chief pharmacist. Other important issues which must be considered when planning the team dynamics include service developments on the horizon, workload volume changes, structural changes in the health service, professional developments and political changes. A chief pharmacist must have a clear vision of team development if he or she is to create a team able to meet its objectives.

Job analysis, job description and personnel specification

Before placing a job advertisement the immediate and future role for the post should be reviewed to ensure an appropriate job description can be written. Table 14.2 illustrates a systematic method for job analysis.

From the job analysis a job description and personnel specification can be written. The job description should describe the job and state the jobholder's responsibilities. Usually the accountability (who manages the post) is stated. There is no standard format, although local standards may be developed in departments or trusts. A personnel specification identifies the characteristics of the jobholder. This includes not only the skills, knowledge, experience, qualifications and attributes needed, but also the

Table 14.2 Checklist for job analysis

High-level questions	The person specification
What is done?	Physical and health requirements
When is it done?	Education and training requirements
Why is it done?	Registration requirements
Where is it done?	Previous experience
How is it done?	General skills and knowledge required
	Communication and interpersonal skills
What are the key responsibilities?	Motivation and leadership skills
Responsibility for staff	
Responsibility for outcomes	**Terms and conditions**
Responsibility for quality	Working environment
Responsibility for finances	Team member or working alone?
	Remuneration, hours, holidays
What are the relationships?	
To whom is the person accountable?	**Testing the results**
What are the key peer relationships?	Check with the current postholder and
Relationships with other departments	with colleagues if the job is designed
Relationships with the public	correctly

personal characteristics that are considered desirable in the successful candidate. A personnel specification will describe the essential minimum standards for the post as well as the desirable qualities that 'better' candidates may have. The purpose is to facilitate shortlisting and appointment, stating objective criteria for the decision-making process. Using this approach can help avoid making poor appointments and ensures that appointments are made on merit rather than personal prejudices.

Advertising

The aim of an advertisement is to ensure a good range of applicants at a reasonable cost. Choice of advertising medium is important: *The Pharmaceutical Journal* is the obvious choice for pharmacist posts, but local papers and in-house magazines are also used. The local paper would usually be the preferred medium for assistant posts. The content of the advertisement should encourage suitable people to apply and discourage those who are not suitable. The information needs to be informative and yet remain clear and concise. Experience dictates that it is essential to proof-read all advertisements before they are finally authorised as agency interpretation can often lead to embarrassing mistakes. A telephone number is normally given through which further information can be obtained. It is advisable that a potential applicant calls to make enquiries regarding a job. This will familiarise the employer with the name of applicants and a little bit about them, which is a useful icebreaker for an interviewee if called for interview. If applying for a position, it can be useful to visit the department and get a feel for the job and the team dynamics. While it is important that the applicant wants to be part of the place, the team and the strategic direction of the department, it is equally important that the department wants the candidate to be part of that team. When the interview stage arrives, candidates should be clear that they will accept the post if they are offered it. It is frustrating for an interview panel to offer a post to a candidate who has decided he or she does not want the job but cannot offer a reasonable explanation.

Application forms

Most hospitals have a standard application form which should be carefully completed. Additional sheets can be added on to the back of these forms for extra supporting information. When a job advertisement generates a large response rate it is easier for the shortlisting team to find all of the information pertaining to an applicant in one place rather than on both the application form and on an accompanying curriculum vitae.

When completing a form, applicants should look at the job description and, if available, the personnel specification and then link their experience and additional information with what is required. They should not simply regurgitate the specification. Many applicants will state that they are self-motivated, enthusiastic and have good organisational or team skills without providing examples of past experience to demonstrate this.

Methods of selection

Most candidates for pharmacy posts will be chosen following an interview. It is often difficult to relax at interview but it is important that the candidate is open and honest so that the panel can assess accurately the personality of the individual and previous experience. An experienced interview panel should help put a candidate at ease and will describe the framework for the interview before it actually starts. If candidates have questions that they wish to ask there is usually time allocated at the end. It is advisable that a candidate makes a list before arriving at the interview as these questions may be forgotten in the pressures of the moment. When preparing for interview there are some standard questions that are often asked and can be anticipated by the candidate. Answers should not simply be regurgitated but some preparation should help the interviewee relax while providing some easy wins. Common questions include:

- Can you give me a summary of your career to date, paying particular attention to the parts of your previous role that are relevant to this position?
- What in particular interests you about this role?
- What can you contribute to the department?

It is important to listen carefully to the questions to ensure that the answers are appropriate, concise and honest and do not meander.

It is now common practice to ask for a presentation to be made, usually at the beginning of the interview. This will help identify the candidate's communication and influencing skills. It is important that the candidate keeps to the allotted time and remembers mainly to discuss the pharmaceutical aspects of the subject as this will be what will interest the panel.

Prioritisation exercises present candidates with a selection of situations which they are required to place in order of priority. It is usual to be able to ask for points of clarification or explanation in these exercises to aid prioritisation, to show that impulsive decisions aren't being made before knowing all the facts.

Sometimes candidates may be invited to meet informally with departmental or other trust staff prior to the interview during what is often described as 'trial by sherry'. This is usually reserved for more senior appointments. For the successful candidate it is the first step towards building relationships with new colleagues.

Psychometric testing is sometimes used in senior management appointments in the hospital. Fortunately for most candidates, the costs and availability of trained personnel needed to administer and analyse the tests limit their use.

Accepting a post

It is important that candidates make the right choice when offered a new position. They should not be pressurised into making a decision quickly if unsure. It is advisable, however, to have researched the post fully before the interview so that a reasonably speedy decision can be made following an offer of employment.

Recruitment and retention

Meeting the current NHS agenda with its ever-expanding roles and opportunities for pharmacy is challenging, especially in the light of the current problems experienced with both the recruitment and retention of pharmacy staff.

The national shortage of pharmacists has left every branch of the profession with vacancies and the hospital sector has had to compete with higher rates of pay in community, industrial and locum pharmacy. Furthermore, the establishment of pharmaceutical and prescribing advice posts in primary care has provided some of the clinical opportunities seen within the hospital sector without the unsociable hours and demanding workload. There is also an increasing shortage of technicians resulting from their expanding roles and the creation of new posts.

Much work has been undertaken across the hospital sector to improve recruitment and retention. Hospitals have more recently started advertising for pharmacists at an undergraduate level. A greater emphasis has been placed on providing vacation work for undergraduates. For some time the extensive undergraduate programme developed by Boots has successfully resulted in the attraction of newly qualified pharmacists into their employment. In many hospitals a training package for vacation students has been established to offer experience in many aspects of the services provided by hospital pharmacy departments. Years ago, vacation students may have been seen as something of a burden or a strain on already stretched resources. Now they are given much greater consideration and more forward-thinking hospitals are enticing them with the opportunity of experiencing clinical work at ward level and spending time in technical services and medicines information. In addition, vacation experience has been elevated to paid work and is no longer seen purely as a valuable experience for the student but rather as an effective recruitment tool for the employer.

In the past, the voluntary nature of this work failed to attract many students for long enough to provide a broad enough experience of the hospital sector and create the desire to return as a graduate. Salaries have now improved for junior pharmacists in an attempt to gain parity between hospital and other branches of the profession. In 1999–2000, a 13% pay rise was awarded to junior grades to reduce salary differentials. But money is not the only determining factor for a newly qualified pharmacist making the choice as to which branch of the profession to enter. Rotational training programmes have been set up to encourage applicants and to improve retention within the hospital sector. As a result many hospitals have developed competence-based training programmes for junior-grade staff and have linked the attainment of competence with progression through the grades. Hospitals, primary care trusts and local community pharmacies have joined forces to offer a wide range of training and experience. Postgraduate courses are now offered routinely as a retention initiative rather than a reward for the exceptional pharmacist. The myth that it is difficult to transfer to the hospital sector once a community or industrial career has been started is being dispelled now and the skills offered by many pharmacists from other branches of the profession are welcomed within UK hospitals. Work is being undertaken by many hospitals to develop accelerated clinical induction packages which will develop the clinical knowledge required for a role in hospital pharmacy while recognising other well-developed and valuable skills.

One of the major attractions of a career in hospital pharmacy is the well-developed roles of support staff. Skill-mix management has progressed over recent years, with technical staff taking on more and more of the non-clinical roles previously held by pharmacists. This is a positive move as it leads to retention of good technical staff and releases pharmacists' time to deal with more indepth clinical issues at a ward level. Dispensaries in some hospitals are run as pharmacist-free zones. Pharmacists are becoming more involved in multidisciplinary team working at ward level, attending ward rounds, giving prescribing advice to medical staff and administration advice to nursing staff and getting involved in aspects of discharge planning such as writing up discharge prescriptions.

Flexible working arrangements are a common feature of hospital pharmacies: job-sharing, part-time hours, career breaks and so on. There is also a growing need to meet the needs of patients and other clinical staff better by providing services beyond conventional working hours.

As well as attracting staff, retaining them is an important part of a manager's role. One aspect of this is to provide a comprehensive induction programme for new appointees. The length and nature of the induction programme will depend on the appointee's experience and post. Typical features will be health and safety information, introduction to colleagues, training on equipment and explanation of procedures and working practices.

Initial induction should be followed up by regular reviews or appraisals. These are opportunities, often on an annual basis, to review performance, celebrate successes, identify training needs and agree objectives or targets for the coming year.

Good communication within a department is important to its effective running and helps retain staff, avoiding uncertainty and involving staff in the changes taking place within the hospital and department.

Misconduct

Ensuring the best staff are appointed, retained and developed are all important roles for the pharmacy manager but occasionally things go wrong. Trusts have disciplinary procedures to deal with misconduct and personnel departments provide help and advice to managers. The first step for minor problems (for example, lateness) will be to counsel the staff member: this is not considered part of the formal process, but does give an opportunity for improvement. Discussion should be confidential, based on evidence and give the member of staff an opportunity to explain his or her viewpoint. Clear timescales, expected standards and review dates have to be specified and agreed with the staff member. If improvement is not achieved or if a more serious matter occurs, the formal steps of the disciplinary policy will be followed. Usually the steps are verbal warning, written warning, final warning, dismissal. However for theft or assault or other very serious acts (usually called gross misconduct) dismissal may follow the first event.

Sickness

On appointment, staff will be reviewed by occupational health staff to check suitability for employment. However, not surprisingly, staff have periods of sickness from time to time. Their manager should be aware of these episodes and ensure appropriate certificates are completed and records made. Support from the hospital's occupational health department can be provided if needed and if repeated periods of sickness occur

Table 14.3   Skills and qualities required by managers

Personal qualities
- Strong leader
- Self-motivated
- Proactive
- Coping with conflicting pressures
- Team player
- Working in a multidisciplinary environment

Skills and abilities
- Presentation skills
- Communication skills – oral and written
- Personal time management
- Analytical skills
- Project management
- Devise, plan and manage complex work programme
- Numeracy and computer-literacy skills

Managing staff
- Individual performance review
- Personal development plans
- Continuing professional development
- Disciplinary procedures
- Workforce planning
- Recruitment and retention

Business planning
- Writing business cases
- Project management
- Budget-setting and management
- Financial skills

Experience
- Evidence of working in relevant settings
- Knowledge of NHS

(three to four in 6 months) a review may be required. Work itself can cause sickness – stress or physical problems – so such causes need to be identified and addressed. Repeated incidents of sickness, with no underlying cause, may result in a similar process to that for dealing with misconduct. When underlying disease or disability is identified as the cause efforts should be made to adapt the job to retain the employee – an aspect of encouraging diversity in the workplace.

Conclusion

The Audit Commission emphasised the importance of the Chief Pharmacist [2]. The growth in spend on medicines and the risks of poor medicines make this importance inevitable. The need for good leadership within pharmacy is a challenge for current and future pharmacy managers. The role of leading a complex pharmacy service in a changing environment is challenging, but seeing success – providing good care, developing people and practice – can be extremely rewarding. Some of the skills needed for the role are listed in Table 14.3.

References

1. Department of Health. *Improving Working Lives for the Pharmacy Team.* London: Department of Health, 2001.
2. Audit Commission. *A Spoonful of Sugar – Medicines in NHS Hospitals.* London: Audit Commission, 2001.
3. Campbell D, Fowler A. Benchmarking: concepts and frameworks. *Pharm Manage* 2001; 17: 52–55.
4. Campbell D, Fowler A. Benchmarking: project planning and implementation. *Pharm Manage* 2001; 17: 56–59.

Further reading

Bee R, Bee F. *Constructive Feedback.* London: Chartered Institute of Personnel and Development, 1998.

Blanchard K, Johnson S. *One Minute Manager.* New York: Harper Collins, 2000.

Department of Health. *Improving Working Lives for the Pharmacy Team.* London: Department of Health, 2001.

Furnham A. *Management Shapers. Body Language at Work.* London: Chartered Institute of Personnel and Development, 1999.

Gareth L. *Mentoring Manager.* London: Institute of Management, 2000.

Gillen T. *Management Shapers. Assertiveness.* London: Chartered Institute of Personnel and Development, 1998.

Maitland I. *Management Shapers. Motivating People.* London: Chartered Institute of Personnel and Development, 1998.

Maitland I. *Management Shapers. Managing your Time*. London: Chartered Institute of Personnel and Development, 1999.

Mumford A. *Management Shapers. Effective Learning*. London: Chartered Institute of Personnel and Development, 1999.

Peters T, Waterman R H. *In Search of Excellence*. New York: HarperCollins, 1995.

15

Support organisations

Jayne Wood and Philippa Jones

The aim of this chapter is to provide information on some of the organisations accessible to undergraduates, preregistration pharmacists and qualified pharmacists working in the hospital sector that can provide professional support, encourage information exchange and enable personal development. The list of organisations is not intended to be exhaustive and it does not cover specialist organisations which may be more relevant to support the advanced pharmaceutical practitioner.

Hospital Pharmacists Group (HPG)

Background

The HPG is a membership subgroup of the Royal Pharmaceutical Society of Great Britain. It considers issues relating to any aspect of hospital pharmacy practice and works to promote knowledge and standards of practice. The group is administered by a committee of 11 pharmacists, two of whom are members of the Society's Council and nine elected members (seven from England, one from Scotland and one from Wales). Membership of the HPG is open to all pharmacists working within the National Health Service (NHS), private or armed forced hospitals and those employed by, or acting as consultants to, health authorities and primary care trusts (PCTs).

Activities

The HPG undertakes a number of activities. It forwards views on policies for development and implementation through the policy support unit to the Society's Council. It advises Council on aspects of hospital pharmacy and health care developments affecting hospital pharmacists and provides HPG members with information about service developments and examples of good practice. It also safeguards the pharmaceutical care of patients by promoting the development and implementation of appropriate standards within hospital pharmacy practice and promoting pharmaceutical skills and knowledge within the hospital service. Further information on the HPG can be found from the Royal Pharmaceutical Society website (www.rpsgb.org.uk).

British Pharmaceutical Students Association (BPSA)

Background

The BPSA, which was founded in 1942, is the national organisation that represents pharmacy students in the UK. It encourages and facilitates the interchange of ideas and opinions between students and represents their views and opinions to the Society and other pharmaceutical bodies. The BPSA also coordinates social and educational events as well as obtaining special discounts and providing services for its members.

Activities

The BPSA holds a number of accredited events, including local educational conferences, competitions at universities and an annual conference. There is also an annual conference for preregistration trainees. It publishes *The Future Pharmacist* [1] for undergraduates and *The Graduate Link* [2] for preregistration trainees as well as providing useful links to assist undergraduates with their course work and careers information on its website (www.bpsa.com).

The College of Pharmacy Practice (CPP)

Background

The CPP, which was established in 1981, is a self-governing organisation of pharmacists who share the aim of promoting and maintaining a high standard of practice. It is committed to continuing professional development (CPD) and it actively promotes an interdisciplinary approach. Its professional development programme is suitable for all pharmacists, whatever their experience or branch of the profession, as it allows individuals to plan and progress their professional development at their own pace.

Current membership comprises over 1550 pharmacists from all areas of the profession. Initially pharmacists join the College as associates by completing an application form and submitting an annual subscription fee. They may then seek full membership either by examination or by practice after completing a portfolio and a supporting submission. Both members and associates are required to provide evidence of at least 30 hours of approved continuing education per year met through attendance at study days, approved courses, participation in Credit for Learning, or completion of relevant distance-learning courses. Members who wish to continue their personal and professional development may then take additional College examinations to attain 100 credits to achieve the Practice Award. Pharmacists also have the option of completing advanced modules, or making a portfolio submission demonstrating their expertise or authority in practice to gain the Advanced Award. Experienced pharmacists who can demonstrate a very high level of practice and achievements at local and national level may also apply for Fellowship, which is the highest award available to College members. There is also an option for pharmacists who have given up full-time practice on a long-term basis for reasons of ill-health, retirement, family commitments or a change of employment into another area of work to apply to become a Friend of the College.

The Continuing Professional Development Portfolio

The Portfolio, which is integral to the Professional Development Programme, enables pharmacists to:

- identify their skills and knowledge
- gain the maximum benefit from formal training and education
- recognise and value workplace training
- record and plan professional development
- express professional aspirations and prepare for College membership by practice and the Advanced Award by Practice (if desired).

Membership by practice

In order to achieve membership by practice associates make a submission, supported by their Continuing Professional Development Portfolio, which demonstrates a high level of practice within their sector of the profession and how their practice meets the following criteria:

- professional growth – the development as a pharmacist over the course of a career
- professional commitment and awareness
- personal CPD
- professional judgement, showing an awareness of legal and ethical matters
- interpersonal and communication skills
- knowledge and understanding of the organisational and policy context within which pharmaceutical services are provided
- an analytical and evaluative approach to practice.

It is expected that at least 3 years' practice experience will be necessary before these criteria can be met. A mentor may be assigned to help with preparation of a submission.

Membership by examination

Associates wishing to use this route to membership must attain 100 credits, of which 60 must be from the following College modules:

- general therapeutics (10 credits)
- practice, law and ethics (10 credits)
- practice scenarios (20 credits)
- practice reports and oral (20 credits)

or

- practice research project and oral (20 credits)

The remaining credits can be made up from either a selection of other College modules, or from approved, externally assessed qualifications. Local study groups and regional facilitators are available to help with preparation for the examinations. Membership by examination is also recognised as part fulfilment of the MSc courses at Aston and Liverpool John Moores universities, and members who achieve 100 credits through college modules are also eligible for the College's Practice Award.

Activities

The College organises approximately six courses every year which cover a number of clinical and managerial topics. Each of these study days is chaired by a College governor and consists of plenary lectures and workshop sessions. The College produces proceedings from these meetings and a number of other publications and reports on a regular basis. These may be purchased from the College.

To support pharmacists there are regional facilitators who act as a local focus for advice and information on the professional activities of the College, particularly in relation to associates preparing for the membership examinations or membership by practice submission. Facilitators also promote College CPD activities, and encourage College members and others to further their CPD and education, and to improve their skills. The College can also provide mentors for pharmacists wishing to pursue membership by portfolio. In addition, the College plays a role in accreditation of courses.

Faculty of Prescribing and Medicines Management

Recognising the development of specialist areas of pharmacy practice, on 15 March 2001, the CPP launched the Faculty of Prescribing and Medicines Management which is a new representative specialist group offering expert advice and support. This first Faculty of the College represents pharmacists from all elements of the profession who provide prescribing advice and/or medicines management support, or who have an interest in this specialist area of practice. The Faculty already has a membership of over 200. The Faculty will strive to ensure that pharmacists working in this specialist area can demonstrate relevant knowledge, skills and flexibility to undertake the range of existing and emergent roles required to meet the challenges of NHS reform. Working to a formal constitution, and under an elected board, the Faculty has defined a range of responsibilities in support of its aims. Developed in consultation with a range of key stakeholders active in this area, the Faculty provides a mechanism by which pharmacists and their organisations can obtain a rapid and informed corporate specialist view on all issues relating to prescribing and medicines management.

The Faculty is an important new professional body that can assist with national strategic thinking, policy development and implementation. In addition, it can offer effective expert and representative input from the membership for any working groups. At the time of writing discussions are underway with other groups regarding the introduction of other specialist faculties.

Further information on the College and its activities can be found from the website (www.collpharm.org.uk).

United Kingdom Clinical Pharmacy Association (UKCPA)

Background

The UKCPA was established in 1981 with the aim of supporting and encouraging the development of clinical pharmacy by bringing together like-minded pharmacists from different practice areas to share knowledge, research and experiences. In 1996, the Association refined and developed this strategy by publishing its *Statement on Pharmaceutical Care* relating to the delivery of pharmaceutical services within the multidisciplinary setting, utilising goals and outcomes agreed with the patient. [3]

Through a programme of conferences, workshops, practice interest groups (PIGs) and publications, the UKCPA encourages the development and evaluation of new services to patients. It offers a supportive network to help pharmacists to enable them to develop, share and exchange ideas, research findings and practical experiences. In this way it encourages pharmacists to refine their skills and develop their level of practice in order to create new and effective working relationships with other disciplines and to engage with the demand for better health care and to meet public health needs.

Current membership comprises over 2000 pharmacists from all areas of the profession. With this broad spectrum of members, the UKCPA is able to access knowledge and expertise in order to examine ways in which pharmacists can deliver patient-focused care. Membership is gained by completing an application form and payment of an annual subscription fee.

Activities

The UKCPA organises two symposia each year in May and November. Each provides a forum for the presentation of research in the form of posters or oral communications. In collaboration with members from the pharmaceutical industry, UKCPA confers awards for original, practice-based research. The symposia are renowned for their interactive and participative workshops which are facilitated by members who are acknowledged experts in their field of practice. The Association also has a number of PIGs. These include:

- antimicrobial management
- critical care
- education and training

- elderly care
- primary care development
- quality assurance
- surgery and theatres.

The aims of the PIGs are to function as a forum for dialogue and exchange of ideas between its own members, as a reservoir of expertise in the field of interest for the organisation as a whole and to promote the field of interest through educational initiatives, workshops and study days. UKCPA also produces a quarterly newsletter. Further information can be found on the website (www.ukcpa.org.uk).

European Society of Clinical Pharmacy (ESCP)

Background

The ESCP is an international body, founded in 1979 by clinical practitioners, researchers and educators from various countries in Europe, which constantly looks for new areas of professional practice. Current membership comprises pharmacists from all areas of the profession within Europe. This includes hospital, community, academia and industry as well as pharmacists working at the interface between primary and secondary care. Since the formation of the Society there has been a gradual and sustained growth of clinical pharmacy in many European countries. The goal of ESCP is to encourage the development and education of clinical pharmacists in Europe. The society tries to achieve its goal by:

- providing a forum for the communication of new knowledge and developments in clinical pharmacy
- promoting the value of clinical pharmacy services among other health care professionals, scientific societies that share the same interest and generally within the NHS
- enforcing the formation of activities in the field of clinical pharmacy and pharmacotherapy through conventions and specific courses
- teaching clinical pharmacy at pre- and postgraduate level
- accrediting centres where clinical pharmacy activities are carried out and which are prepared to host visiting pharmacists or pharmacy students
- promoting multicentre research in all areas of clinical pharmacy
- promoting the participation of pharmacists in clinical trials
- producing a number of publications on clinical pharmacy
- promoting a more widespread use of existing clinical pharmacy publications.

Activities

ESCP holds a symposium on clinical pharmacy every autumn. At this forum, which includes plenary lectures, moderated discussions, round-table discussions and workshops, clinical pharmacy practitioners from various countries have the opportunity to meet and exchange knowledge and experience about new developments in clinical pharmacy. There are also oral communications, poster discussion forums and poster presentations. Special interest groups organise their annual meetings dedicated to specific fields of clinical pharmacy. Among others, cancer care, medicines information, geriatrics, nutritional support, paediatrics and pharmacoepidemiology are prominent. ESCP also organises a spring conference, which is focused on a specific theme to provide professional education.

On the day prior to the annual symposium, ESCP organises a masterclass in 'Search of Excellence', which is dedicated to a specific topic related to the special interest groups. ESCP also offers awards to individual researchers in clinical pharmacy fields in collaboration with sponsors. A number of accredited centres have been established to enable European clinical pharmacists to gain experience in a range of clinical pharmacy specialities. ESCP has also produced a database of clinical pharmacy courses in Europe.

ESCP edits and issues journals, including the scientific journal *Pharmacy World and Science* [4], where research papers and proceedings of the annual symposium are published. The ESCP newsletter, which is published bimonthly, serves as a link between the Society and its members, and provides news about its activities as well as the activities of its members. In addition ESCP selects existing clinical pharmacy publications for promotion to members of the Society.

Related organisations

To promote the value of clinical pharmacy services among other health care professionals and scientific societies, ESCP has established a relationship with societies which share the same interests. These include the American College of Clinical Pharmacy (ACCP), European Association of Hospital Pharmacists (EAHP), European Pharmaceutical Students' Association (EPSA), Royal Dutch Association for the Advancement of Pharmacy (KNMP) and the UKCPA. ESCP has also been recognised by the Efficacy Working Party of the European Agency for the Evaluation of Medicinal Products (EMEA) as a contributor in the consulting process. Within the European Forum of Pharmaceutical Associations and the World Health Organization regional office for Europe (EuroPharm Forum), ESCP is appointed as observer organisation. Further information on ESCP can be found on the website (www.escp.nl).

Centres for Pharmacy Postgraduate Education

Background

There are four centres for pharmacy postgraduate education – the Centre for Pharmacy Postgraduate Education in England (CPPE), the Scottish Centre for Post Qualification Pharmaceutical Education (SCPPE), the Welsh Centre for Postgraduate Pharmaceutical Education (WCPPE) and the Northern Ireland Centre for Postgraduate Pharmaceutical Education and Training (NICPPET). Each centre has a slightly different role, which will be described below.

Activities

CPPE (England)

Established in 1991, the centre is based at the University of Manchester and its aims are to plan and coordinate the provision of continuing education for community pharmacists in England. The programme has recently been extended to include pharmacists working in the hospital sector.

The mission of CPPE is to implement a programme of professional postgraduate education, to meet national and local needs, to increase participation and develop opportunities for pharmacists to respond to changes in pharmacy practice. Led by a team based at the university, continuing education is provided by distance-learning materials in varying forms and face-to-face learning through workshop sessions. A large network of local pharmacy tutors is responsible for facilitating continuing education activities at local level. Priority topics are decided by the national Steering Committee on Pharmacy Postgraduate Education (SCOPE), which takes account of:

- the Royal Pharmaceutical Society's national continuing education syllabus for pharmacy (core syllabus) (published in the *Medicines, Ethics and Practice Guide* [5] which is sent to all pharmacists)
- future roles of the community pharmacist

- policy initiatives from the Department of Health, for example key areas identified in the *Health of the Nation* [6].

In addition local needs can be incorporated through the input of the local tutor. Workshop material and distance-learning materials are prepared by experts working within a project team in a particular subject, commissioned by the CPPE. Prospectuses are circulated on a quarterly basis. Further information can be found on the website (www.cppe.man.ac.uk).

SCPPE (Scotland)

The Post Qualification Education (PQE) board for Scottish pharmacists was established following an extensive review by the Scottish Office Home and Health Department (SOHHD). The main functions of the PQE board are to advise on the education and training needs of NHS pharmacists in Scotland, and to oversee the organisation of courses to meet those needs by effective and efficient means. The organisation of course provision in Scotland is undertaken by SCPPE, based in the School of Pharmacy at the University of Strathclyde. SCPPE aims to maximise the contribution of community and hospital pharmacists in the NHS in Scotland through the provision of appropriate postqualification education and training programmes. Its objectives are to:

- ensure that the programme of education and training activities meets the requirements of current professional, scientific and practice developments
- provide refresher courses for pharmacists wishing to return to pharmacy practice
- develop and apply indicators of quality and performance to ensure that courses meet their stated objectives and to report on these to the PQE board
- minimise overlap of course provision and accreditation procedures and maximise the utilisation of available expertise and other learning resources
- assist in the development of educational methods.

Coordinated by staff based at SCPPE, there is a network of local tutors and national tutors who organise courses for all NHS pharmacists in Scotland. Continuing education is provided by three main methods:

- direct-learning courses
- distance-learning packages
- sponsorship for postgraduate diploma/degree courses – most are in clinical pharmacy.

The SCPPE syllabus is provided from the 5-year rolling programme of continuing education for NHS pharmacists in Scotland. The 40 topic areas in the rolling programme are divided into three main areas:

- disease management
- personal and professional development
- health promotion.

Further information can be found on the website
(www.scppe.strath.ac.uk).

WCPPE (Wales)

The Welsh Committee for Professional Development in Pharmacy
(WCPDP) was the successor to the Welsh Committee for Postgraduate
Pharmaceutical Education. The Committee oversees the development of
a broad range of education-related support for pharmacists and qualified
support staff in Wales which is provided by the WCPPE.

WCPPE is based within the Welsh School of Pharmacy in Cardiff;
its aims are to develop and deliver a broad range of education-related
support for pharmaceutical staff in Wales. The Deputy Director organises a programme of courses for hospital pharmacists and also a series of
residential courses for hospital-based preregistration graduates. A team
of full-time tutors develop core continuing education courses for community pharmacists throughout Wales. A support staff coordinator
organises courses for qualified support staff (BTEC technicians or equivalent) and also runs the Welsh Pharmacy National Vocational
Qualification (NVQ) Centre through which WCPPE can accredit NVQ
courses and NVQ assessors. It is increasingly common for courses to be
organised for mixed audiences of participants from the staff groups
described above, thus allowing the support of the whole pharmaceutical
team. In addition to providing face-to-face and online courses, the Centre
coordinates a free video-loan library for use by pharmacy staff in Wales
and distributes a range of distance-learning packs. Further information
can be found on the website (www.cf.ac.uk/phrmy/wcppe).

NICPPET (Northern Ireland)

NICPPET provides CPD to pharmacists and other health care professions in Northern Ireland. Its mission is 'to support through education
and training a quality pharmaceutical service'.

Based at Queen's University Belfast, the centre coordinates learning programmes based on workshops, distance-learning packages,
open-access evening courses or online training. NICPPET also operates

a library loan service and the website offers a literature-searching facility. Prospectuses for the learning programmes are circulated to pharmacists twice a year. Further information can be obtained from the website (www.nicppet.org or www.qub.ac.uk/pha/nicppet).

Guild of Healthcare Pharmacists (GHP)

Background

The GHP was founded in 1923 (originally as the Guild of Hospital Pharmacists). It is the independent voice representing the interests of hospital pharmacists in professional matters and in negotiations on salaries and conditions of employment. Membership of the Guild is open to all practising hospital pharmacists in the UK and members participate in the work of the Guild through local groups which conduct professional, business and social meetings throughout the year. Membership is gained following completion of an application form. Fees are paid monthly by individuals or through their employer.

Activities

Policies at national level on professional and non-professional matters are decided by a council of 22 members who are elected by the membership. Guild Council is supported by four main committees – practice, education and science, organisation, and terms and conditions. There is also an international committee and an executive committee. The executive committee meets for ad hoc executive functions between Council meetings as required by the President.

In 1974, in order to provide the professional negotiating skills needed within the Pharmaceutical Whitley Council, where salaries and conditions of service are decided, the Guild merged with the Association of Scientific, Technical and Managerial Staff (ASTMS). This union later became MSF (Manufacturing, Science and Finance) following merger with another union (Technical, Administrative and Supervisory Staffs, or TASS). The Guild, through its Council and general membership, retains a clear identity and independence within MSF. The services of MSF are available to the membership, including representation in the event of difficulty in the work situation, legal support where appropriate and educational facilities. The staff-side of the Pharmaceutical Whitley Council is nominated by the Council of the Guild: the Chair is a member of Guild Council and the Secretary is a full-time officer of MSF.

The GHP is active in promoting the profession of hospital pharmacy. Several scientific awards are available to members by competition and these are administered by the Education and Science Committee of the Guild. *Guild News* is regularly mailed to the membership free of charge and the Guild is regularly commissioned to contribute papers and articles to the *Pharmaceutical Journal* on all aspects of hospital pharmacy. Professional events such as the weekend school, day conferences and symposia are organised each year providing the opportunity for pharmacists to present work undertaken as a result of a Guild award, such as a travelling fellowship. Guild Council nominates representatives to 14 British Standards Committees and is consulted on all relevant draft documents from various official and professional bodies which interface with the profession. Further information can be found on the website (www.ghp.org.uk).

References

1. www.bpsa.com/services.php?page = future_pharmacist   (accessed   13 November 2002).
2. www.bpsa.com/services.php?page = grad_link (accessed 13 November 2002).
3. www.ukcpa.org/default.asp?channel_id = 447&editorial_id=1819   (accessed 20 November 2002).
4. Anonymous. 30th European symposium on clinical pharmacy integrating pharmaceutical care into practice. *Pharm World Sci* 2002; 24: 17–39.
5. *Medicines, Ethics and Practice*, 26th edn. London: Royal Pharmaceutical Society of Great Britain, 2002.
6. Department of Health. *The Health of the Nation: A Strategy for Health in England*. London: HMSO, 1992.

Further reading

British Pharmaceutical Students Association website. www.bpsa.com (accessed 13 November 2002).

Centre for Pharmacy Postgraduate Education in England (CPPE) website. www.cppe.man.ac.uk (accessed 13 November 2002).

College of Pharmacy Practice website. www.collpharm.org.uk (accessed 13 November 2002).

European Society of Clinical Pharmacy website. www.escp.nl (accessed 13 November 2002).

Guild of Healthcare Pharmacists (GHP) website. www.ghp.org.uk (accessed 13 November 2002).

Royal Pharmaceutical Society website. www.rpsgb.org.uk (accessed 13 November 2002).

Scottish Centre for Post Qualification Pharmaceutical Education (SCPPE) website. www.scppe.strath.ac.uk (accessed 13 November 2002).

United Kingdom Clinical Pharmacy Association website. www.ukcpa.org (accessed 13 November 2002).

Welsh Centre for Postgraduate Pharmaceutical Education (WCPPE) website. www.cf.ac.uk/phrmy/wcppe (accessed 13 November 2002).

Index

Page numbers in bold indicate main discussion; numbers in *italic* refer to figures and tables

accelerated clinical induction packages, 248
Accident and Emergency (A&E)
    prescribing for patients, 38
    violence to staff, 179
acute hospital trusts, 6, *8*, 12–13
acute pain management, 135
additives, intravenous, preparation, **61**
Administration of Radioactive Substances Advisory Committee (ARSAC), 67
administrative staff, *12*
Advanced Award, CPP, 255
adverse drug reaction (ADRs), **127–128**, 131
    reporting, 128, 181
adverse event reporting, **182–183**
advertising
    direct-to-consumer (DCA), 131
    jobs, **244–245**
advisory services, quality assurance, 81
Agenda for Change, 12
AIDS/HIV, **138**
air pressure differential monitoring, 86
air velocity measurements, 86
airborne subvisual particle counting, 86
Aitken Report, 30
ambulance trusts, 2, *8*
amino acids, administration, 140
anaesthetics, supply to
    dentists, 194
    theatres, 138
Analytical Information Centre (AIC) database, 77
analytical methods, QC laboratories, 83–84

annual budget, hospital trusts, 238
annual reports, hospital trusts, 176
annual trend data, 241
antibiotic infusions, domiciliary patients, 61
antibiotic resistance, 157
anticoagulant services, **133–134**
antipsychotics, 142
application forms, staff, **245–246**
Application of the Medicines Act to Health Authorities, 73
Aseptic Dispensing for NHS Patients, 61
aseptic preparation, 47, **60–67**
    facilities and equipment, **63–66**
    the future, 69, 70
    history, 49
    process, **66–67**
    quality assurance, 66–67, 73–74, 80–81, 87
        environmental monitoring, **86–87**
        laboratories, quality control testing, 85
        quality audit, 81
        research and development, 82
    scope, **60–63**
        cytotoxics, **62–63**
        intravenous additives, **61**
        radiopharmaceuticals, 63
        total parenteral nutrition (TPN), *62*, *64*, *65*, 140
    training, 65, **67–68**
assistants, *12*, 146, 193
    job advertisements, 244
    training, **229**
Association of the British Pharmaceutical Industry, 176

Association of Scientific, Technical and
Managerial Staff (ASTMS), 264
attitude measurement, 218
audit, 174, 175, 183
definition, **211**
professional and clinical, **132–133**
quality, **81**
Audit Commission
A Spoonful of Sugar, xviii, **xx**, 13,
80, 145, 154, 168, 225, **241**
chief pharmacist influence, 9
CIVAS use, 61
definition, medicines management,
172
formularies, 158
information technology usage,
203, 209
innovations in practice supported
by, *146*
outpatient dispensing, 38
purchasing of medicines, 27
robotic systems, 44
audit trail, 33, 38, 122
autoclaves, 58, *59*, 60
automation, **208–209**
dispensing systems, 146, 208
repackaging, 52, *53*
robotic system handling, 43–44, 208
in sterile manufacture, 58
Automix system, TPN compounding,
64, *65*
awards
College of Pharmacy Practice (CPP),
255
Practice Research, RPSGB, 219
Galen, 219
Sir Hugh Linstead Community
Research Fellowship, 219

bar code scanning, **43, 209**
basic-grade pharmacists, *13*
batch documentation, 26, 57
BCG programme, 197
bedside medicines cabinet, 30, 31, 32,
34, **35–36**
automated, 208
controlled drugs (CDs), 41
benchmarking, 175, **240–243**

NHS Benchmarking Reference
Centre, 18
performance indicators, criteria used,
242
*Better Information for Managing
Medicines*, 94
bibliographic databases, 115
black triangle medicines, 158
blood products, 26
boards, hospital trust, 8–9, 154–155,
156
Boots undergraduate programme,
247–248
branded medicines, 18, 19
Breckinridge Report, 49, 61
Bristol inquiry, 175
British National Formulary, 157, 176
nurse prescribing, 192
British Pharmaceutical Students
Association (BPSA), 254
budget management, 234, 236
drug budget, **239–240**
staff budget, **238–239**
Building a Safer NHS for Patients, 76
bulk solutions, preparation, 58
history, 48–49
bulletins, 195
medicines information, 101
prescribing messages, 163
business case
developing for new drug, 159
preparing, **237**
business planning, **236–237**
Buttercups scheme, 228

Cadbury Committee, corporate
governance report, 171
capital funding, 236, 237, 238
care, levels of, *3*
Care Standards Act (2000), 198
care trusts, xvii, 5, 201
career pathways, 12, *15*
case-control studies, **217–218**
Centralised Intravenous Additive
Services (CIVAS), 47, 49, 60, 61
Centres for Pharmacy Postgraduate
Education, 227, **261–264**
background, 261

CPPE (England), **261–262**
NICPPET (Northern Ireland),
    263–264
SCPPE (Scotland), **262–263**
WCPPE (Wales), **263**
charities, research funding, 219
chemistry facilities, quality control
    laboratories, **83–85**
Chief Administrative Pharmaceutical
    Officers, Wales, standards
    document, xviii
chief pharmacist, 9, 11, *13*, 29, 224,
    234–236, 251
    annual business plan, 236–237
    budget management, **238–240**
    strategic management, 235
chromatography, high-performance
    liquid, 83–84
chronic pain management, 135
clean areas, environmental monitoring,
    86–87
cleaning procedures, repackaging
    equipment, 54
clerical staff, *12*
clinical audit, 133, 175
clinical benchmarking, *see*
    benchmarking
clinical effectiveness, improving,
    175–176
clinical governance, 75, 81, **175–177**,
    212, 224, 234
    definition, **212**
    in medicines information, **99–104**
    pharmacy's role, 177
clinical guidelines, prescribing advice,
    163, *164*
clinical negligence scheme for trusts
    (CNST), **184**
clinical pharmacy, 104, **121–146**, 182,
    223
    the future, **145–146**
    history, 122
    medicines management, definition,
    121
    pharmaceutical care, 125, 127
    roles for clinical pharmacist, *126*
    pharmaceutical care activities
    anticoagulant services, **133–134**

concordance, **130–131**
education and training others, **132**
increasing role of technician,
    135–136, 146
medication errors and ADR
    reporting, **127–128**
medication history taking,
    128–129
medicines formularies
    development, **132**
outpatient clinical pharmacy
    services, **134**
pain management, **135**
patient education and counselling,
    129–130
pharmacokinetics and therapeutic
    drug monitoring, **131–132**
prescribing advice, **127**
prescription monitoring, **126–127**
primary/secondary care interface,
    134–135
professional and clinical audit,
    132–133
self-administration schemes, **131**
prescribing, moving into, xx, 138,
    143–145
services linked to medical specialities,
    136–143
critical care, intensive care and
    theatres, **139**
general medicine and elderly care,
    136–137
HIV/AIDS, **138**
mental health, **142–143**
nutrition, **139**, 140
    see also total parenteral
    nutrition (TPN), aseptic
    preparation
oncology, 140, *141*
    see also cytotoxics
paediatrics, 140, *141*
renal services, **141–142**
surgery, **137–138**
ward pharmacy, **121–122**
clinical risk, 151, 157, **180–184**
clinical trial certificate (CTC), 41, *42*
clinical trial exemption certificate
    (CTX), 41, *42*

clinical trials, **41–42**, 87, 174
  drug manufacture, 58, 74
  medicines information, *98*
  trial protocol, pharmaceutical input,
    173
Clinical Trials Directive, 213
clinician, definition of, 125
CLINTIS computer system, 42
closed questions, 218
Cochrane database, 216
cohort studies, 217, **218**
College of Pharmacy Practice (CPP),
    254–257
  activities, **256–257**
  background, **254–255**
  Continuing Professional
    Development Portfolio, 255
  Faculty of Prescribing and Medicines
    Management, **257**
  membership by examination, **256**
  membership by practice, **255–256**
combined trusts, *8*
Commission for Health Improvement
    (CHI), **178**
commitment contracts, 21
Committee on Safety of Medicines,
    128
common drug file, 205, 206
  see also standard drug database
community health services (CHS), 187,
    188, 190
  services provided, *189*
Community Services Pharmacists
    Group, 188, 197
community services pharmacy,
    187–201
  advice, **190–191**
  developments in prescribing and
    administration of medicines,
    191–192
  dispensing for hospital outpatients,
    xvii, 37
  education and training, **195–196**
  elderly care, **198**
  the future, **200–201**
  history, **187–190**
  information, **195**
  learning disabilities, **199**

  monitoring safe practices with
    medicines, **196**
  public health programmes,
    supporting, **196**
  residential and nursing homes,
    197–198
  school nursing, **196–197**
  supply, **192–195**
  working with other agencies,
    199–200
community trusts, 2, *8*
competency, 117, **227–228**
Competition Act, 25
complaints, **176–177**
compliance, 128
computer systems, 155–156
  clinical trials administration, 42
  invoicing, 27
  stock control, 25–26, 155–156, 203,
    204–205, 205–206
  see also electronic prescribing
concordance, 128, 129, **130–131**
confidentiality, *98*, 181
confounding, observational studies, 217
consequences, clinical risk, 180
Conservative government, 2
containers
  non-sterile manufacture, 57
  sterile manufacture, 58
continuing education, 228, 230
  definition, *226*
continuing professional development
    (CPD), 177, 226, 230
  Continuing Professional
    Development Portfolio, CPP,
    255
  definition, *226*
  QC laboratory staff, 85
contraceptives, 193
contracting
  contracting cycle, *23*
  EU directives, 20
  first hospital contracts, **18–19**
  offer evaluation and negotiation
    within process, **21**
  organisation, hospital contracts,
    22–24
  procedures, **20–21**

review of performance, 19–20
strengths of contracting process, **22**
types of contract, **21–22**
*Control of Substances Hazardous to
    Health* (COSHH), 68, **179–180**
controlled drugs (CDs), **39–41**
    administration/supply, 40
    disposal, 40
    goods receipt, 27
    storage, 31, **40–41**
        cupboard keys, 31
Controls Assurance Standards,
    171–173, 225, 234
    medicines management, 29,
        172–173, 193
copyright, 99
coroners, medicines information, 99,
    105
corporate governance, 171, 234
costs
    electronic patient records (EPR), 207
    hospital prescribing, *153*, 160
        impact of clinical pharmacists on,
        165
    new drug, 158, 159
    primary care prescribing, 152, *153*
    staff costs, dedicated outpatient
        pharmacy, 38
    see also expenditure, medicines
counselling patients, **129–130**, 137
critical appraisal, research articles, 216
critical care, clinical pharmacy, **139**
critical incident reports (CIRs), 101,
    182, 183, 184
cross-contamination, avoiding, non-
    sterile preparations, 57
cross-sectional surveys, 218
Crown immunity, loss of, 50
Crown Review, **143–144**, 213
cupboards, medicines storage, 31
    controlled drugs (CDs), **40–41**
    keys to, 31
cytotoxics, 180
    aseptic preparation, **62–63**, 140
    process, 66, 67

DARE (Database Abstracts of Reviews
    of Effectiveness), 216

data protection, *99*
The Data Protection Act (1984), 213
data sheets, COSHH regulations,
    179–180
day-case patients, medicine supply, 38
defamation, *98*
defective medicines, 83, 84
degree courses, 225
dentists, supply to, **194**
Department of Health, 4
    Enterprise Scheme, 213
dependent prescribers, 144
    see also supplementary prescribing
deregulating medicines, 131
diaries, research, 218
direct-to-consumer advertising (DCA),
    prescription medicines, 131
directorate drug budgets, 239
directorate pharmacists, **163**, 239, 240
directorate structure, hospital trusts,
    9–10, **10–11**, 156
    influencing prescribing at corporate
        level, 162–163
Directorates of Health and Social Care,
    7
discharge medication, 34, **35**, 36, 51,
    208
    writing orders for, 143
discharge planning, 137
disciplinary procedures, 249–250
disclaimers, *98*
    handling of PODs, 35
disinfectants, COSHH regulations, 180
disposal
    controlled drugs (CDs), **40**
    patients' own drugs (PODs), 35, 40
    unused clinical trial drugs, 42
dissemination of research, 219–220
distance learning, 228
district general managers, 2
district health authorities, 2
district management teams, 1–2
district nurses, supply to, **194–195**
district pharmaceutical officers, 187,
    197
district prescribing committee, 161
district prescribing groups, 160, 161,
    165–166

divisions, clinical, 9, 156
doctor or dentist exemption certificate
  (DDX), 41, *42*
dose monitors, 65
dose-banding, cytotoxics, 63
drug alerts, 83
drug allergies, 138
drug budgets, **239–240**
Drug Information Services, 92
  see also medicines information (MI)
drug interactions, 131
Drug and Therapeutics Committee,
  154, **155**, **158–160**
  formulary contents, 157–158
Drug Therapy and Pharmacy, 213
dust extraction systems, 52
Duthie Report, 40, 193

education authorities, working with,
  200
education and training, **223–230**
  community health staff, **195–196**
  the future, **229–230**
  history, **223–225**
  hospital technical services, **67–68**
  management and leadership, **229**
  medical, pharmacist contribution to,
    183
  pharmacists, **227–228**, 248
    clinical pharmacy, **132**, 227
    medicines information services,
      116–118
    undergraduate and preregistration,
      224, **225–226**
  in quality assurance, 82
  support staff, **229**
  technician training, 224, **228–229**
  see also patient education and
    counselling
elderly care, **136–137**
  intermediate and continuing care
    services, **198**
  residential and nursing home
    inspection, **197–198**
electrolytes for TPN feeds, 58
electronic data interchange (EDI), 26,
  43, 203, **204–205**
electronic invoice files, 27

electronic patient records (EPR), 27,
  156, 176, 204, **206–208**
electronic prescribing, 118, 137, 146,
  183, 204, 206, **207**, 209
Embase, 115
endotoxin testing, 85
English Regional Pharmaceutical
    Officers, standards, xviii
enquiry answering, medicines
    information, 100–101, **106**, *107*
  technician responsibility, **117–118**
enuresis clinics, 187
environmental issues, technical services,
    68
environmental monitoring, 66, **86–87**
epidural infusions, 61
errors, reporting of, 127–128, 182–183
ethics
  and legal issues, medicines
    information, 95, **96–97**, 97–99
  in research, **218**
ethics committees, 218
  clinical trials, 41
European Society of Clinical Pharmacy
    (ESCP), **259–261**
  activities, 260
  background, **259**
  related organisations, **260–261**
European sources, research funding,
    219
European Union (EU) legislation and
    hospital procurement, **20–22**, 25
  background and requirements, **20**
  types of procedure, **20–21**
evidence-based practice, **175–176**
executive board members, hospital
    trusts, 8, 9
exemption documents, clinical trials,
    41, *42*
expenditure, medicines, 17, 151, 152,
    153, 160, 205, 238
  management of, 239–240
  reports to trust management boards,
    154, *155*
  see also costs
experimental studies, 216, **217**
extemporaneous dispensing work, 55, 80
external medicine cupboards, 31

Faculty of Prescribing and Medicines Management, CPP, 257
family planning clinics, supply to, **193**
family practitioner committees, 2
Farillon, vaccines supply, 193
faxing orders, 26
Fellowship of College of Pharmacy Practice (CPP), 255
filter integrity testing, 86
financial implications, paediatric drug therapy, 141
financial risk, **151–152**, 157, 171
financial systems data, 156
fire procedures, 178
A First Class Service: Quality in the New NHS, 4, 75, 99, 174, **175**, 177, 224
definition of clinician, 125
flexible working arrangements, 249
formularies, **132**, **157–158**, 176
nurse prescribers formulary, 192
foundation hospitals, 13
FP10(HP) forms, 37, 38
framework contracts, **21–22**, 23
funding
capital, 236, 237, 238
for research, **219**
The Future Pharmacist, 254

Galen Award, 219
Gateways, 216
gene therapy, 63, 68, 87
general management, 2
general managers, 11
general medicine, clinical pharmacy, **136–137**
general practice
family practitioner committees, 2
fundholding, 2–3
practices within PCO, 5
general practitioners (GPs)
advice to, xvii
shared-care agreements, 37, **161–162**
vaccines supply to, 193
generic errors, testing for, 182
A Generic Perspective, 19–20
generic substitution, **18**, 19
gluteraldehyde, 180

good manufacturing practice (GMP), 75, 78, 79
goods receipt, **26–27**
grades and roles
pharmacists', *13*, 227
technicians, *14*
The Graduate Link, 254
Griffiths Report, 2
Guidance Note 14, 50
Guidelines for Registration and Inspection of Private Nursing Homes, 197
Guild of Healthcare Pharmacists (GHP), 227, **264–265**
research funding, 219
Guild News, 265

Health Act (1999), 3, 4
health authorities, 1, 2, 4, 5
strategic, 7
health boards, Scotland, 6
health circulars
HC(84)3, 49, 73
The Way Forward, **xix-xx**, 124
Health Memorandum HM(65)22, 73
health and safety, **178–179**
technical services, **68**
health service research (HSR), definition, **211**
Health and Social Care Act (2001), 145
Health and Social Services Secretary, Wales, 4
Health Technical Memorandum (HTM2022), 82
health visitors, supply to, **195**
Hepler and Strand, concept of pharmaceutical care, 125
high-efficiency particulate air (HEPA) filters, testing, 86
high-performance liquid chromatography, 83–84
HIV/AIDS, **138**
homogeneity, finished products, 57
hospital manufacturing, *see* technical services
Hospital Pharmacists Group (HPG), 34, **253–254**

hospital pharmacy, definitions and functions, **xvii-xviii**
hospital trusts, 2, **8–9**, 50
  annual budget, 238
  annual reports, 176
  business planning, **236–237**
  clinical negligence scheme for trusts (CNST), **184**
  example of structure, *10*
  pharmacy's place in, **10–11**
  staffing budget, **238–239**
  trust management board, 8, 9, 156
    and prescribing issues, **154–155**

illegal substances, disposal, 40
immunisation
  school vaccination programmes, **196–197**
  staff, 179
  vaccines supply to GPs, **193**
Improving Health in Wales, 212
in-house training programme, 226, 227
independent prescribers, 144
individual patient dispensing, 30, **33**
individual patient supply, **33–37**
  non-stock dispensing, **33**
  one-stop dispensing, **34**
  patients' own drugs (PODs), **34–36**
  unit dose systems, 30, 35, **36–37**, 40, 121, 131, 138
individualised TPN feeds, 62
induction programmes, new appointees, 249
  accelerated, 248
infections, 157
informal networks, developing, 11
information
  provision of, community services pharmacists, **195**
  use of, **176**
    see also medicines information (MI)
information resources, **114–115**
information technology, **115–116**, 118, **203–209**
  automation, 208–209
  electronic data interchange (EDI), **26**, 43, 203, **204–205**

electronic patient records (EPR), 27, 156, 176, 204, **206–208**
electronic prescribing, 118, 137, 146, 183, 204, **206**, 209
  history, 203–204
  stock control systems, 155–156, 203, 204–205, **205–206**
inpatient dispensing, **31–37**, 42–43
  individual patient supply, **33–37**
  ordering ward stock, **32–33**
  storage arrangements, **31–32**
instrumental methods of analysis, 83
integrated-care pathways, 176
intellectual property rights (IPR), hospital-developed formulations, 50, 69–70
intensive care units, clinical pharmacy, **139**
interface, primary/secondary care, **134–135**
intermediate care beds, elderly people, 198
internal market, 2–3
internal medicine cupboards, 31
international sources, research funding, 219
internet, 94, 176
  medicines information, 114, 115, 131
  patient safety site, 206
interviews
  job applicants, 245, **246**
  in research studies, 218
intranet, 115, 183
intrathecal administration, cytotoxics, 67
intravenous additives, aseptic preparation, **61**
intravenous nutrition (IVN), *see* total parenteral nutrition (TPN), aseptic preparation
invoicing, 27
ISO 9000 quality system model, 86
ISO/IEC 17 025 standards, 86
isolator systems, 63, 65
  air exchange monitoring, 86

job
  advertising, **244–245**

analysis, 244, *245*
description, **244**

labelling, 51, 52
  checking against master, 57
laboratory services, quality control, 73,
    77, 79, **83–86**, 87
Labour government, 1, 3, 224
laminar air flow cabinets, 58, 63, *64*
  air exchange monitoring, 86
lead time, 26
leadership, 229, 234–236
learning disabilities, support for, **199**
learning disability trusts, *8*
legal and ethical issues, medicines
    information, **95**, 96–97,
    97–99
legal representatives, medicines
    information, 99
licensing issues, 4, **50–51**
  clinical trials, 41–42
  specials licence, **50–51**, 57, 61, 78,
    79, 84
lifelong learning, 177, 224
  definition, *226*
likelihood, clinical risk, 180
Likert scale, 218
Linstead report, xvii-xviii, 152
liquids
  non-sterile production, 54, 56
  repackaging, 54
  sterile production, 59
literature search, 214, 216
local education authorities, working
    with, **200**
local health groups, Wales, 6
local papers, job advertisements, 244
local research ethics committee (LREC),
    218
locum staff, 239
longitudinal surveys, 218
loss-leading, avoiding, 158
lymph scanning, 63
lyophilised powders, parenteral
    formulations, 60, **61**

macronutrients, 140
main group contract, 23

managing services, **233–251**
  benchmarking, 18, 175, **240–243**
  budget management, **238–240**
    drug budget, **239–240**
    staff budget, **238–239**
  business planning, **236–237**
    preparing business case, 237
  pharmacy management, **234–236**
  skills required by managers, *250*
  staff management, **243–251**
  training, **229**
manpower planning, 241, 243
manual handling, 178–179
manufacturer's specials licence, *see*
    specials licence
Manufacturing, Science and Finance
    (MSF), 264
mass immunisation campaigns, 197
measles/rubella immunisation, 197
the media, medicines information, 99,
    105
Medical Devices Agency, 4
medical gases, testing installations, **82**
Medical Research Council, 219
  clinical trial guidelines, 41
medical technical officers (MTOs), *12*
  see also technicians
medical training, pharmacist
    contribution to, 183
medication errors, **76**, 80, **127–128**,
    145, 209, 241
  reducing, 30, 76
    physician order entry, EPR, 206
    repackaging schedule, 54
    robotic systems, **44**, 208
    unit dose systems, 36–37
medication history taking, 127,
    128–129, 136–137
Medication Management course,
    technicians, 229
Medicines Act (1968), Section 10,
    unlicensed products, **50**, 61
Medicines Control Agency, 4, 50, 79,
    174
  Defective Medicines Reporting
    Centre, 83
  Guidance Note 14: 69
  inspections, 61, 86

Medicines, Ethics and Practice – A Guide for Pharmacists, 95, 96–97
medicines information (MI), 91–119, 195
  activities, 105–112
    proactive, 106, 107–108, *109–112*
    reactive, 106, *107*
  aims and strategy, 93, 94–95
  clinical governance and risk management, 99–104
  customers/users, 104–105
  ethics and legal issues, 95, 96–97, 97–99
  the future, 118
  history, 91–92
  information resources, 114–115
  information technology, 115–116, 203–204
  to medical and nursing staff, 127
  roles and skills, 95, *96*
  specialist information services, 113–114
  staffing and training, 116–118
  structure, 92–93
medicines management, *see* Audit Commission *A Spoonful of Sugar*; pharmacy management; strategic medicines management
Medicines Management Controls Assurance Standard, 29, 172–173, 193, 234
  Controls Assurance criteria October 2001, *173*
Medicines Management Framework self-assessment, 158
Medicines Management Group, North Staffordshire Hospital Trust, 155
Medicines Management (MM) Collaborative, 220–221
Medicines, Pharmacy and the NHS: Getting it Right for Patients and Prescribers, 213
Medicines Review Group, **166**
Medline, 115
meningitis C vaccination, 197
mental health, clinical pharmacy, 142–143

mental health trusts, 8
methodology, research project, 216–218
MI-UK, e-mail discussion group, 116
microbiological contamination
  minimising, sterile products, 59
  non-sterile raw materials, 57
microbiological monitoring, 86–87
microbiology facilities, QC laboratories, 85
microfiche databases, 204
micronutrients, 140
middle-grade pharmacists, *13*
misconduct, **249–250**
Misuse of Drugs regulations, 27, 39
Misuse of Drugs (Safe Custody) Regulations 1973, 40
Modern Laboratory Information Management Systems (LIMS), 85
Modern Materials Management (MMM) Consultancy Group report, **19**
monoclonal antibody products, 87
MSF (Manufacturing, Science and Finance), 264
multicentre research ethics committee (MREC), 218
multicompartmental TPN bags, 62
multidisciplinary working, 196

National Care Standards Commission, 198
national competency framework, MI, 117
national development scheme for senior pharmacists, 229
National Electronic Library for Health (NeLH), 95
National Institute for Clinical Excellence (NICE), 94, **166–167, 174–175**
National Introductory MI Training Course, 116
National Patient Safety Agency (NPSA), 76
National Pharmaceutical Association (NPA), 228

National Pharmaceutical Supplies
  Group (NPSG), 24
National Prescribing Centre, 108, 156
National Purchasing and Supply
  Agency (NPSA), 27
National Service Frameworks, 175
  for older people, 137, 198, 200
National Vocational Qualification
  (NVQ)
  Level 2, pharmacy assistants, 229
  Level 3 in Pharmacy Services, 228
  Welsh Pharmacy NVQ Centre, 263
negative-pressure isolators, 63
negligence and liability, 97
  clinical negligence scheme for trusts
    (CNST), **184**
negotiated contracting procedure, 21
new drugs, 157–160, 166
  D&T committees, **158–160**
  formularies, **157–158**
  new product scheme, 108
    stage 1 and 2, new drugs in
      research, *109–110*
    stage 3, new drugs in clinical
      development, *111*
    stage 4, new medicines on market,
      112
The New NHS: Modern, Dependable,
  3, 5, 174
new procedures, publicising, 183
news sheets, 183
newspapers, job advertisements, 244
NHS Benchmarking Reference Centre,
  18
NHS and Community Care Act (1990),
  2
NHS Direct, 94, 105
NHS Executive Letters EL(96)95 and
  EL(97)52, 74, **81**
NHS executive (NHSE), 4
  performance management, 6
  regional offices, 3, **4**
NHS, hospital pharmacy within, **1–15**
  the future, 12, 13
  history, **1–4**
  the new NHS until 2002, **4–5**
  NHS hospital trusts, **8–10**
    pharmacy's place in, **10–11**

The NHS Plan, 7–8
  see also The NHS Plan
Northern Ireland, 6–7
pharmacy staff, **11–12**
primary care organisations,
  evolution, **5–6**
Scotland, 6
Wales, 6
NHS hospital trusts, *see* hospital trusts
NHS National Horizon Scanning
  Centre, 108
NHS National Prescribing Centre, 108,
  156
NHS Pharmaceutical Quality Control
  Committee, 77, 78, 87
The NHS Plan, xx, 4, 7–8, 12, 17–18,
  87, 192, 212
NHS Quality Control Committee, 81
NHS reforms
  impact of, **19**
  influence on strategic medicines
    management, **165–166**
NHS Supplies, 19, 20
  see also Purchasing and Supply
    Agency (PaSA)
NHS24, 105
NICE, *see* National Institute for
  Clinical Excellence
no-smoking policy, 179
Noel Hall report (1970), xviii, **xix**, 2, 92
non-executive board members, hospital
  trusts, 9
non-sterile manufacture, **54–57**, 68–69
  facilities and equipment, **55–56**
  history, 48
  process, *57*
  scope, **54–55**
non-stock dispensing, **33**
Northern Ireland
  health care, 4, **6–7**
  NICPPET, **263–264**
Notified Body inspection, 86
NSF, *see* National Service Frameworks
nuclear medicine, 63, 67
  see also radiopharmaceuticals,
    preparation
Nuffield Report (1986), **xix**, 122, 124,
  152

nurse prescribing, **191**, **192**, 194, 195
nurse requisitioning, **32–33**
nursing homes, **197–198**
nutrition, clinical pharmacy, **139**, 140
   see also total parenteral nutrition
     (TPN), aseptic preparation

observation charts, 127
observational studies, 216, **217**
occupational health department, 250
on-call clinical trials team, 42
oncology, clinical pharmacy, 140, *141*
   see also cytotoxics: aseptic
     preparation
one-stop dispensing, **34**
open contracting procedure, 20–21
open questions, 218
operating department practitioners, 39
operational management, 235
operator protection testing, 86
Orange Guide, *see Rules and Guidance*
    for Good Pharmaceutical
    Manufacture and Distribution
ordering medicines, **25–26**
   controlled drugs (CDs), **39**
   electronic data interchange (EDI), **26**,
     43, 203, **204–205**
   ward stock, **32–33**
     ward order assembly agreement,
      43
An Organisation with a Memory, 76,
    181, 207
Our Healthier Nation, 4
out-of-date resources, 115
outpatient dispensing, xvii, **37–38**, **134**
outreach pharmacy services, 134
over-the counter medicines, 131

pack sizes, range of, 208
paediatric medicines, 54–55, 61, **140**,
   141
pain management, 135
palliative care, subcutaneous infusions,
   61
parallel-imported medicines, 25
parenteral nutrition, 139, 140
   see also total parenteral nutrition
     (TPN), aseptic preparation

participatory observation, 217
patient education and counselling,
   129–130, 137
patient group directions (PGDs), 143,
   191
patient information leaflets (PILs), 34,
   105
patient medication records, 205
   see also electronic patient records
     (EPR)
patient packs, 34, 51
patient representative
   involvement in service quality
     assessment, 177
   NHS trust boards, 9
patient-controlled analgesia, 61
patients' own drugs (PODs), **34–36**,
   121, 131
   disposal, 35, 40
   perioperative period, 138
patient's perspective, hospital
    pharmacy, xviii
patients, questioning, 127
pay
   junior pharmacist improvements, 248
   modernisation, 12
performance management framework,
   152, **153–154**
performance reviews, staff, 249
performance standards, 225
perioperative period, PODS, 138
permit-to-work system, 82
personnel specification, **244**
pharmaceutical care
   clinical pharmacist roles, *126*
   components of delivery, **126–136**
   concept of, 125
pharmaceutical companies, 17–18, 219
Pharmaceutical Interlaboratory Testing
    Scheme (PITS), 86
The Pharmaceutical Journal, 244, 265
Pharmaceutical Price Regulation
    Scheme (PPRS), **17–18**, 25
Pharmaceutical Society of Great
    Britain, 92
   see also Royal Pharmaceutical
     Society of Great Britain (RPSGB)
Pharmaceutical Whitley Council, 264

pharmacist prescribing, xx, 138, **143–145**
Pharmacist and the Profession, 213
pharmacokinetics, **131**
Pharmacy in the Future (2000), **xx**, 8, 87, 152, 208, 225
Pharmacy In A New Age (PIANA), 213
pharmacy management, **234–236**
Pharmacy Practice: Setting the Research Agenda: Self-care and Pharmacy, 213
pharmacy practice research (PPR), **211**
Pharmacy in Scotland, 212
pharmacy tendering evaluation (PHATE), 24
PhD studentships, 219
physician order entry, EPR, 206
piped medical gas installations, testing, 82
pneumatic conveying (air tube) systems, 43
podiatrists, supply to, 194
police
  advice from, CD storage, 41
  medicines information, 99, 105
Post Qualification Education (PQE) board, Scotland, 262
post registration courses, 224
postal ordering, 26
'postcode prescribing', 167, 174
postgraduate courses, 132, 227, 248
potassium chloride ampoules, storage, 41
Practice Award, CPP, 255
Practice Research Awards, RPSGB, 219
preadmission clinics, 129, **138**
prepacked medicines, 38, 43, **51**
  see also repackaging (prepacking, assembly)
preregistration training, 224, **225–226**, 230
prescribers, influencing, **162–165**
  at corporate level, **162–163**
  individual prescribers, **163**, **164–165**
prescribing
  advice to medical staff, **127**
  electronic, 118, 137, 146, 183, 204, 206, **207**, 209

nurses, **191**, **192**, 194, 195
pharmacists, xx, 138, **143–145**
supplementary, 192
prescribing costs, 152, *153*, 160
  impact of clinical pharmacist on, *165*
prescribing issues, senior management awareness of, **154–155**
prescribing reports, 154–155, 156
prescription charges, 1
  clinical trial patients, 42
prescription sheets, 30, 122, *123*, 127
prescriptions, 39
  average per head, 151
  review and monitoring, 30, **126–127**, 127, **137**, 164, 206
presentations at interview, 246
primary care, *3*
  formularies, 158
  prescribing costs, 152, *153*
  staff, involving in hospital D&T committees, 159, 161
primary care groups (PCG), 3, 5, 104, 160
primary care organisations (PCOs), **5–6**, 7
primary care trusts (PCTs), xvii, 3, **5**, 7, 94, 158, 160, 166, 188, 189, 190
  medicines information services usage, 105
primary/secondary care interface
  clinical pharmacy, **134–135**
  discharge planning, 189–190
  strategic medicines management, **160–161**
prioritisation exercises, 246–247
private hospitals, storage of CDs, 40
private sector, research funding, 219
proactive information, *98*, 101
professional self-regulation, **177**
protocols, clinical trials, 42
provider trusts, 2, 6, *8*
  see also hospital trusts
psychometric testing, job applicants, 247
public health programmes, supporting, **196**
public sector, research funding, 219
purchasers and providers of care, 2
  see also provider trusts

purchasing group contracts, 22–23, 24
purchasing medicines, 17–27
 background, 17–18
 the future, 27
 goods receipt, 26–27
 history, 18–20
 hospital procurement and EU
  legislation, 20–22
 invoicing, 27
 ordering, 25–26
 organisation, hospital contracts,
  22–24
 quality assurance, 79
 recent changes, 25
 strengths of contracting process, 22
 systems and processes, 24
Purchasing and Supply Agency (PaSA),
 19, 22
 management systems, 24
 working relationship with, 24

qualitative research, 217, 218
quality assurance, 73–88
 advisory services, 81
 aims of NHS quality assurance
  services, 76–77
 of aseptic services, 66–67, 73–74,
  80–81
 defective medicines, 83
 development, issue, implementation
  and monitoring of standards, 78
 environmental monitoring services,
  86–87
 the future, 87–88
 laboratory services, 83–86
 medicines information services, 101,
  102
 NHS quality agenda, 74–76
 of pharmacy services, 79–80
 piped medical gas installations,
  testing, 82
 quality audit, 81
 and quality control of medicines,
  78–79
 research and development, 82
 training staff, 82
*Quality Assurance of Aseptic
 Preparation*, 64, 80

quality control (QC)
 during tendering process, 24
 laboratory services, 73, 77, 79,
  83–86
 of medicines, 78–79
 sterilisation processes, 60
  history, 49
quality controller, 81
quality in NHS, 174–178
quantitative research, 217, 218
quarantine, sterile products, 60
quasiexperimental studies, 217
questionnaires, survey, 218

radiopharmaceuticals, preparation, 63
 audit, 81
 facilities and equipment, 64, 65
 history, 49
 process, 67
 workstation, 66
radiopharmacy, on-site, 67
radioprotection, 65, 179
rapid response procedures, defective
  medicines, 83
record keeping
 clinical trial drugs, 42
 controlled drugs (CDs), 39
recorder level, stock items, 25, 26
recruitment and retention, staff,
  247–249
reflective practice, 230
 definition, 226
refrigerators, lockable, 31
regional health authorities, 1, 3, 19
regional MI centres, 92
regional offices, NHS executive
  (NHSE), 3, 4
Regional Pharmaceutical Officer,
  standards, xviii
regional quality control (QC)
  laboratories, 73, 79
 databases, 77
Registered Homes Act, 197
registers, controlled drugs, 39
renal services, clinical pharmacy,
  141–142
repackaging (prepacking, assembly),
  51–54

facilities and equipment, 52, *53*
process, **52, 54**
scope, **51–52**
requisition books, 33, 39
research and development, **211–221**
definitions, **211–212**
the future, **220–221**
history, **212–213**
project design, **214–220**
decision tree, *215*
dissemination, **219–220**
ethics, **218**
funding, **219**
literature search, **214**, 216
methodology, **216–218**
research question, **214**
quality assurance and control, 82, 84
see also clinical trials
research governance, 220
A Research Governance Framework for
Health and Social Care, 220
residential and nursing homes, **197–198**
Resource Discovery Network, 216
resources, medicines information,
114–115
restricted contracting procedure, 21
Review of NHS Pharmaceutical
Contracting, NPSA, 27
The Right Medicine: A Strategy for
Pharmaceutical Care in
Scotland, xx
risk management, **75–76, 171–184**
clinical risk, **151**, 157, **180–184**
history of risk, 181–182
risk action, **183–184**
controls assurance, **171–173**
medicines management, 172–173
COSHH regulations, 68, **179–180**
financial risk, **151–152**, 157, 171
health and safety, **178–179**
medicines information services,
102–103
standards, *103–104*
quality in NHS, **174–178**
see also quality assurance
risk-free medicines, **180–181**
robotic systems, handling patient packs,
43–44, 208

root cause analysis, 182
Royal Pharmaceutical Society of Great
Britain (RPSGB), 227
clinical governance framework,
99–100
clinical trials guidelines, 41
Hospital Pharmacists Group (HPG),
253–254
one-stop dispensing, 34
legal aspects, controlled drugs, 39
Pharmacy In A New Age (PIANA),
213
pharmacy practice research (PPR),
213
research funding, 219
training standards, 225
Rules and Guidance for Good
Pharmaceutical Manufacture
and Distribution, 55–56, 64
quality assurance, 74, 75

safety profiles, 158
salaries, *see* pay
Saving Lives: Our Healthier Nation, 196
school nursing
vaccination programmes, **196–197**
vaccines supply, **193**
Scotland
GPs and transfer of clinical
responsibility, 37
health boards and provider
organisations, 6
hospital outpatients, dispensing for,
xvii
SCPPE, **262–263**
The Right Medicine: A Strategy for
Pharmaceutical Care in
Scotland, xx
Scottish parliament, 4
search engines, 216
secondary care, *3*
Secretary of State for Health, 4
Section 10 exemption, Medicines Act,
50, 61
security measures, 30, 31
self-administration schemes, 31, **32**, 34,
121, **131**
controlled drugs (CDs), 41

self-care, *3*
self-help groups
  medicines information, 105
  working with, 200
self-regulation, professional, 177
senior pharmacists, *13, 29*
  see also chief pharmacist
serial numbering, 33
Service and Financial Framework
      (SAFF) process, 236
shared-care agreements, 37, **161–162**
shelf-life, radiopharmaceuticals, 63
Shifting the Balance of Power
      documents, 7
short-line stores, 19
sickness, staff, 178, **250–251**
Sir Hugh Linstead Community
      Research Fellowship, 219
skill-mix, 241, 248–249
skills training, 183
small-scale non-sterile manufacturing,
      56
smoking, no-smoking policy, 179
social services, working with, **199–200**
solid-dose repackaging line, *52, 53, 54*
special assembly licence, repackaging,
      52
specialist sterile product units, 49,
      57–58
specialists, technical and procurement,
      24
specials licence, **50–51**, 57, 61, 78, 79,
      84
A Spoonful of Sugar, see Audit
      Commission *A Spoonful of
      Sugar*
stability studies, 84
  UK Stability Database reports, 77, 82
staff, **11–12**
  assistants, *12*, 146, 193, 229, 244
  budget, **238–239**
  chief pharmacist, *see* chief
      pharmacist
  costs, dedicated outpatient
      pharmacy, 38
  education and training, *see* education
      and training
  immunisation, 179

  medicines information service,
      116–118
  QC laboratory, 85
  shortage of, 241, 247
  skill-mix, 241, **248–249**
  technicians, *see* technicians
  violence to, 179
staff management, **243–251**
  accepting a post, **247**
  advertising, **244–245**
  application forms, **245–246**
  job analysis, job description and
      personnel specification, **244**, *245*
  methods of selection, **246–247**
  misconduct, **249–250**
  sickness, 178, 179, **250–251**
  recruitment and retention, **247–249**
  selection strategy, **243–244**
standard drug database, 204
  see also common drug file
standards, **xviii**, 174
  aseptic preparation, 80
  controls assurance, 29, **171–173**,
      234, 293
  development, implementation and
      monitoring of, 78
  laboratory QC work, 85–86
  medicines information services,
      100–101
    minimum information resources
      standard, 114–115
    risk management, *103–104*
  performance, 225
Steering Committee on Pharmacy
      Postgraduate Education
      (SCOPE), **261–262**
sterile manufacture, 57–60, 68–69
  facilities and equipment, **58**
  history, 48–49
  process, **59–60**
  scope, **57–58**
sterilisation cycle, 59, 60
sterilisers and monitoring equipment,
      58
stock
  clinical trial drugs, 42
  goods receipt, **26–27**
  ordering, **25–26**

controlled drugs (CDs), **39**
  ward, 31, **32–33**
stock control systems, 155–156, 203,
  204–205, **205–206**
turnover rate, 18
storage of drugs, 30, **31–32**
  controlled drugs (CDs), 40–41
strategic health authorities, 7
strategic management, 235, 237
strategic medicines management,
  151–168
  clinical risk, **151**, 157, **180–184**
  external influences on, 165–167
  financial risk, **151–152**, 157, 171
  history, **152–154**
  influencing prescribers, **162–165**
  information and financial issues,
    155–157
  new drugs, medicines policy
    management, **157–160**
  primary–secondary care interface,
    160–161
  procurement of medicines, **160**
  senior management awareness,
    154–155
  shared care agreements, **161–162**
  see also Audit Commission *A*
    Spoonful of Sugar
structured interviews, 218
structured observation, 217
subcutaneous infusions, palliative care,
  61
substitution, generic, 18, 19
supplementary prescribing, 192
suppliers
  authorising payment, 27
  performance, 26
supply of medicines, **29–44**
  clinical trials, **41–42**
  to community health services,
    192–195
  controlled drugs in hospital, **39–41**
  the future, **42–44**
  history, 30
  to inpatients, **31–37**, 137
  to outpatients, xviii, **37–38**, 134
support organisations, **253–265**
surgery, clinical pharmacy, **136–137**

survey studies, 216, **218**
suspensions, repackaging, 54
systematic reviews, 216

targeted therapy, 63, 68
Task and Finish Group on Prescribing
  Report, Wales, xx, 38
teachers, medicines administration, 200
teaching hospital trusts, *8*
Technical, Administrative and
  Supervisory Staffs (TASS), 264
technical services, **47–70**
  aseptic preparation, 47, 73–74,
    60–67
  education and training for, **67–68**
  the future, **68–70**
  health and safety and environmental
    issues, **68**
  history, **48–50**
  licensing issues, **50–51**
  non-sterile manufacture, 48, **54–57**,
    68–69
  repackaging (prepacking, assembly),
    51–54
  sterile manufacture, **57–60**, 68–69
technicians, 11, *12*, 163, 224, 230
  clinical pharmacy role, **135–136**,
    146
  grades, *14*
  medication history taking, 128
  medicines information service,
    117–118
  medicines supply to community
    health services, 193
  senior management positions, 235
  shortage of, 247
  technician checking schemes, 228
  training, 224, **228–229**
technology appraisals, NICE, 174
telephone helplines, information
  services, 105
tertiary (and higher) care, 3
theatre, clinical pharmacy, 136–137,
  139
therapeutic drug level monitoring
  (TDM), **131–132**
'therapeutic explosion', 92
top-grade pharmacists, *13*

topical preparations, production,
54–55, 57
history, 48
total parenteral nutrition (TPN), aseptic
preparation, **62**, 140
Automix system for compounding,
64, *65*
total quality management (TQM), 74
training, *see* education and training
Treaty of Rome, 20
trend data, 241
trolleys, ward medicine, 30, 32
trusts, 2, 12, 188
business planning, **236–237**
clinical negligence scheme for trusts
(CNST), **184**
hospital trusts, *see* hospital trusts
primary care trusts (PCTs), *see*
primary care trusts (PCTs)
tube-filling and sealing equipment, 56
tutor assessments, 226

UK Accreditation Service (UKAS),
standards compliance, 86
UK CIVAS group, **60**, 69
UK Clinical Pharmacy Association
(UKCPA), 219, **258–259**
UK Medicines Information Pharmacists
Group (UKMIPG), 92, 97, 100
UK Medicines Information (UKMI), 92
UK Stability Database, 77
UK Standard Clinical Products
Reference Source Project
(UKCPRS project), 206
undergraduate training, **225**
vacation work, 247–248
unit dose systems, 30, **36–37**, 208
unit general managers, 2
Unit for Health Services Development
contracting arrangements report,
19–20
unlicensed medicines
medicines information, *98*
production of, 50, 79, 87
see also specials licence
unstructured interviews, 218
user involvement, service planning,
177

vacation work, undergraduates,
247–248
vaccination programmes, school
nursing, **196–197**
vaccine supplies for GPs, **193**
validity, research, 217
Value for Money Unit, 18
VAT on medicines, 17, 37
verbal ordering, 26
violence to staff, 179
viral vectors for drug delivery, 68
visual display units (VDUs),
monitoring, 179
voluntary agencies, working with, **200**
see also charities, research funding

waiting time, hospital dispensing, 38
Wales
Chief Administrative Pharmaceutical
Officers, standards document,
xviii
health authorities, local health
groups and NHS trusts, 6
National Assembly, 4
*Task and Finish Group for
Prescribing Report*, xx, 38
transfer of prescribing, 37
WCPPE, **263**
Welsh Committee for Professional
Development in Pharmacy
(WCPDP), 263
Welsh Pharmacy National Vocational
Qualification (NVQ) Centre, 263
walk-in centres, 196
Wanless Report, 206
ward medicine trolley, 30, 32
ward order assembly agreement, 43
ward packs, 48, **51**
ward pharmacists, 30, 163
ward pharmacy, **121–122**, 223
ward rounds, pharmacist attendance,
127, 164, 165
ward stock, ordering, 31, **32–33**
topping up, 33
ward storage of drugs, 31, 32
controlled drugs (CDs), **40–41**
The Way Forward, health circulars
(1988), **xix-xx**, 124

websites
British Pharmaceutical Association
(BPSA), 254
College of Pharmacy Practice (CPP),
257
European Society of Clinical
Pharmacy (ESCP), 261
Gateways, 216
medicines information, **115–116**
Royal Pharmaceutical Society, 39,
254
Technical Specialist Education and
Training (TSET), 68

United Kingdom Clinical Pharmacy
Association (UKCPA), 259
weighing areas, non-sterile
manufacture, 55
wet analysis, 83
whole-time equivalent posts (WTEs),
238, 239, 241
workload, 240–243

Yellow Card scheme, 128, 181